Your Breath is Your Power

Dramatically improve your health, running, fitness and sport.

First Edition

Jason Kelly B.S.
Exercise Physiologist

If you would like to contact me about lectures, seminars, workshops or further education, please contact me at:

tbblife.com

Visit this website for video and further support about the concepts in this book.

Your Breath is Your Power
Dramatically improve your health, running fitness and sport.

Cover Images by: Jason Kelly and Karla Patricia Barbosa Kelly
Interior Photos by: Karla Patricia Barbosa Kelly

First Edition
First Printing, July 2016

Printed in the United States of America

TABLE OF CONTENTS

Preface

"The beginning is the most important part of the work." –Plato

In order to achieve maximal health, performance and endurance: in order to have the greatest amount of strength, power, fitness, vitality, energy and stamina, you need to breathe functionally and well. This book will teach you the importance and how to breathe through your nose to use your diaphragm. From the general to the athletic population, breathing through the mouth produces fatigue and disease and less endurance, strength and power. When you use the diaphragm to breathe, it produces intra-abdominal pressure. Intra-abdominal pressure produces tension that develops the core and the abdominals stability and strength. The stability and strength developed by the core and the abdominals; is used by the spine to attain stability and alignment in life and for functional movement and mobility. It is the key in developing maximal strength and power for fitness and sport because breathing ramps up the nervous systems power that increases the power in the core to be transferred through movement. During your strength or fitness sessions, you should be getting stronger in your sets and reps, especially in the third set. If not, then you are not using your breath properly for training.

When people train, they fail to train strength without coordinating and integrating breathing into movement patterns, poses, exercises or even into life. Once your breathing is fatigued, limitations and compensations take place. When breathing through the nose you fill the lungs fully from top to bottom. In contrast, breathing through the mouth uses only the top of the lungs. Therefore, you are losing about 50% of your potential to increase your volume of oxygen and straining the lungs because you are not breathing properly. The strength and size of your muscles do not matter when you are sucking wind through your mouth. The person who can breathe well and move functionally and efficiently in their sport or performance has the most cardiovascular stamina, physical power and potential. Life, fitness and sport functions best when it is sustainable to perpetuate longevity and growth. Breathing is the gas for everything: to maintain and enhance training, sports, health and energy to survival. It needs to be as functional and productive as possible. When it is not, it can be the answer to being tired as well as the limitation hindering progression. How you breath will determine health, strength and performance.

Breathing through the nose affects and integrates the respiratory, cardiovascular, musculoskeletal and nervous system. So, when you run, jump, punch, kick, throw, tackle, push or pull, etc., breathing is the platform, the foundation, that integrates and strengthens all the systems together to perform. You need to be mindful of your breathing and train it into your health and fitness program to make it habitual so it becomes highly effective.

All of the aforementioned above cannot be achieved from breathing through your mouth. It does the exact opposite, hampers energy, potential and performance.

Introduction

"Look deep into nature and you will understand everything better." – Albert Einstein

Learn how breathing through your nose and mouth is the difference between:

- Health and disease.
- Sub par strength and maximal power.
- Becoming an athlete and a champion.

Breathing diaphragmatically:

- Produces the proper function and capacity of O_2 (oxygen) and CO_2 (carbon dioxide) balance and exchange in the lungs. You need CO_2 to attract oxygen.
- Through the nose contains a special gas that cleans and warms the air as well as acts as a vasodilator for veins and arteries. Vasodilation means that veins and arteries stay dilated, open. This will enhance performance. The mouth cannot do this and will do the opposite, constrict, and leads to disorder and disease.
- Produces the pressure and tension needed to form the core and produce abdominal stability for spinal alignment.
- Provides power to contact muscles more powerfully and to be flexible instantly.
- Ramps up the (CNS) central nervous systems power.
- Increases strength and power for fitness and athletic performance.
- Creates energy, vigor, vitality, stamina and endurance.
- Will create better health and life.
- Is the anti-aging formula to maintain and re-establish youth.

Chapter 1
Your Breath Is Your Power
"Natural forces within us are the true healers of disease." – Hippocrates

The power of breathing is unconscious to us. It is automatic and involuntary. We don't think about it. Breathing just happens making us less aware of how it is functioning. Often we do not pay attention to whether we are breathing deep or shallow or through the nose or mouth. The only way to know is to be mindful of breathing, to feel it and train it into performance or daily life. What we feel is what truly activates mindfulness and its functions, not what we can consciously see. *Your breath is your power.* Breathing affects every aspect of the mind, body and spirit.

Life, health, youth, vitality, longevity, exercise and movement all depend on how you breathe. The failure to get breathing to regulate respiratory and cardiovascular demands first limits health and progression. When less efficient and effective, the body makes more effort through force and overtraining that nonetheless end up being subpar. Such results are primarily due to breathing through the mouth and not training the diaphragm by breathing through the nose. This is a big issue in health and fitness today. People work and train harder than they can functionally breathe, hoping that it will make all their fitness dreams come true overnight. This is far from the truth. Once your breath becomes shallow during exercise, it's just a matter of time before you need to stop.

Let's look at running as an example. People try to run faster than they can actually breathe. The demand for oxygen becomes higher than the lungs can supply and the level of carbon dioxide (CO_2) is rising. The brain reacts by increasing the breathing rate to inhale more oxygen, hence, resorting to mouth breathing. If you can't maintain breathing through your nose and start sucking wind through your mouth, then you're running too hard, not meeting the level of demands produced by running—your training level is too high. Breathing through your mouth, sucking wind and panting causes your postural muscles to weaken and creates a rounded spine because of the lack of pressure and tension generated to produce stability from the core and abdominals. Breathing through the mouth into the top of the lungs will improve your training somewhat but will be limited in progression because of dysfunction and compensation. When you allow the compensation of breathing through the mouth, you create physical joint compensations and disrupt the levels of CO_2 leading to the constriction in veins, arteries and muscles, and therefore, you affect performance and health. Mouth breathing is neither an efficient nor qualitative way to breathe because of breathing into a smaller space (the top of the lungs) where there is limited capacity and alveoli to do it. Mouth breathing uses more breaths and energy per breath than one breath of nasal diaphragmatic breathing. If you run slower and focus on breathing through the nose using the diaphragm (tame the ego and don't assume that faster is better in the beginning), you will increase the amount of oxygen you take in and create stability for the joints, core and spine effectively, producing energy efficiency. When you run faster, you breathe faster but you need to train yourself to breathe in deeper and longer through the nose to regulate the demands being produced. At rest and during exercise, breathing through the nose is a longer breath that equals more volume, more capacity, less strain and lower heart rate. Breathing through the mouth is a shorter breath that equals less volume, less capacity, more strain and a higher heart rate because of dysfunction.

Over the years from teaching people how to strength train and run, most of them did not breathe correctly or well, providing the explanation of why they could not increase running endurance and why they were experiencing pain. After training and improving their breathing, all those people could run better, longer and experienced less fatigue. Even at rest they felt less fatigue in their recovery. They also started to become more mindful when running. They knew that when they felt fatigue to breathe deeper and to make sure that they were breathing through the nose to do it. This helped them run longer using their natural functional breathing pattern to manage their respiratory system effectively (relaxation mode) instead of breathing through the mouth. During running, if you are mindful of your breathing, you will prevent breathing through the mouth and the inhibition it produces against your performance.

With so much power, why is nasal diaphragmatic breathing underrated, undertrained and not practiced often by everyone? There are many breathing practices and methods. Some are simple and some are advanced in their training. The most important thing for you to do is always start simple and master simplicity to be functional. As you master simplicity, you will build a strong foundation on which you can construct strength methods because it will provide structure, function and efficiency for progression. Without structure you can't make additions to support expansion. Without function you lose the integrations that produce movement, efficiency and its practicality. The loss of efficiency develops more strain and force. Forcing works against natural development. Therefore, you lose your functional ability.

Remember: All training and performance is about training your breath. You become what you train and train what you become.

BREATHE WITH YOUR NOSE,
EAT WITH YOUR MOUTH

We are born breathing through the nose and eating with our mouth. Stress and the modern lifestyle have switched, compensated and evolved our breathing pattern to the mouth.

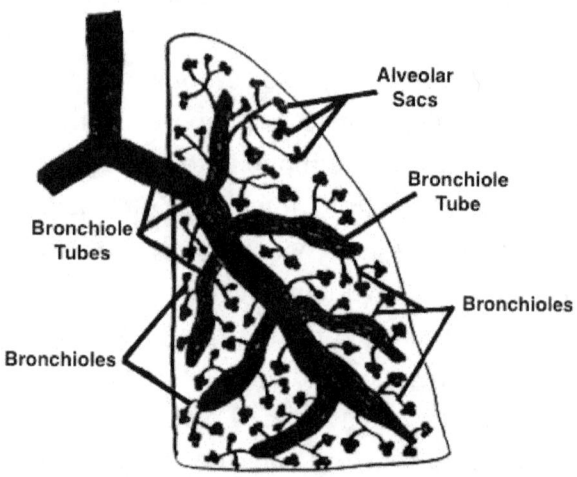

As you inhale air, it flows through the bronchial tubes and through the bronchioles (the smaller branches that ramify from the tubes) where the oxygenated air reaches the alveolar sacs.

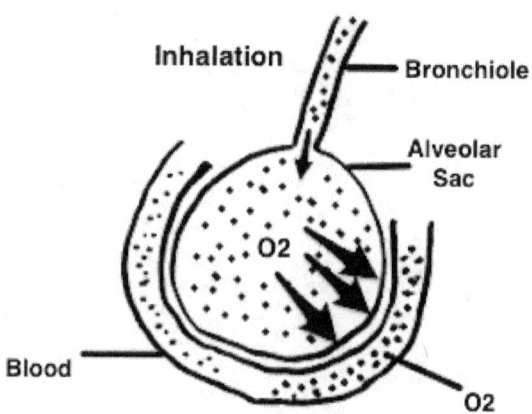

As oxygen enters the sacs, it goes through the capillaries, where it then, enters the blood.

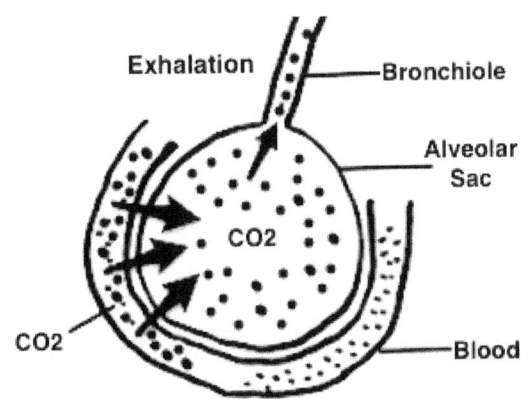

When you exhale CO_2 exits the blood via the capillary entering the alveolar sacs moving through the bronchioles where CO_2's final path goes through the larger bronchial tubes and out of the nose or mouth.

How we breathe is crucial to our health, fitness and performance. There are two different ways to deliver oxygen to your lungs– through your mouth and your nose. Mouth breathing is inhaling and exhaling through your mouth into the top of lungs. It is not very effective because the lungs are narrower at the top of the chest where there is less space and capacity in comparison to the lower area of the lungs. The top spaces of the lungs don't expand like the bottom of the lungs because the diaphragm is not used effectively through mouth breathing. Using only a small amount of surface area in the upper lungs in comparison to the larger spaces in the lower lungs produces strain that leads to dysfunctional breathing. When breathing through your mouth into a smaller surface area, it produces shorter and shallower breaths that increase the breathing rate. Increasing the breathing rate makes the heart work harder and faster to pump blood, producing a higher heart rate.

On the other hand, nasal diaphragmatic breathing (NDB) is inhaling through the nose. It contracts and flattens the diaphragm from its dome shape. NDB counteracts all the dysfunctional issues that mouth breathing produces. Which is why when people start to breathe through the nose, breathing problems and issues diminish and subside. When the diaphragm contracts, it pulls down the bottom of the lungs, increasing the size of the lungs about three times the size of the upper lungs. From the photos, **Inhalation and Exhalation,** you can clearly see there is more surface area in the lower lungs than in the upper lungs containing vast amounts of alveoli to exchange O_2 and CO_2 in the bottom during inhalation. In one nasal diaphragmatic breath you can increase about 30 to 50 percent more O_2 and CO_2 exchanges than one mouth breath because of the diaphragm contracting and expanding the lungs, increasing the capacity in the lower lungs instantly. This results in breathing less and a lower heart rate taking strain off the lungs and heart.

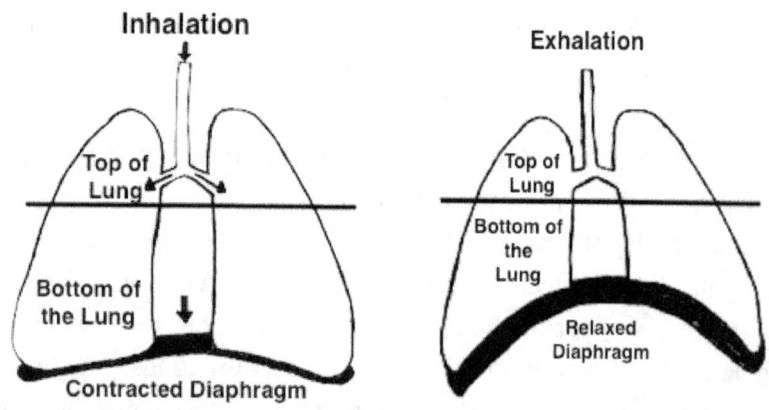

Lower area = more surface area = more exchanges = no strain, relaxed.

Upper area = less surface area = less exchanges = strain, forcing the lung.

WHY WE NEED CO$_2$

The amount of CO_2 that exits the lungs is very important because you do not want to clear all the CO_2 out of your body. How we release it, through the nose, pursed lips or an open mouth, is pivotal. Breathing through the mouth produces an imbalance between O_2 and

CO_2 quickly. You can breathe in and out more **liters of air quicker** in one breath through your mouth than your nose. But just because it's faster and does more, does not make it better. It produces dysfunction. Although you can inhale and exhale more air through your mouth, there is a very small percentage of O_2 that gets inhaled and perfused because mouth breathing causes CO_2 levels to remain low. When you exhale through the mouth it releases too much CO_2 that produces imbalance. The nose is a better system to control airflow.

• **Inhaling as much air as you can, taking in many deep breaths through your mouth, does not mean you are increasing the amount of O_2 in your body.** It is the exact opposite. If CO_2 levels are low in the blood then O_2 will not be released or inhaled. If your body does not need oxygen or it is not exchanged properly then it is just a wasted breath. A wasted breath consumes energy and produces strain on the heart. Breathing through the mouth at rest or during exercise, exhales too much CO_2 at one time, making the levels drop too quickly, creating O_2 deficit and deficiency. It is a big reason why muscles get tight and constricted at rest, during exercise, fitness and sports performance because of poor regulation. It is a big reason why fatigue sets in quicker because blood flow is constricted. The large amounts of CO_2 exhaled through the mouth produces an alkaline condition in the blood that constricts arteries and veins affecting the brain and the heart as well as the muscles decreasing the cardiovascular and musculoskeletal systems performance. When CO_2 levels fall, O_2 is held and not released from the blood. It is why the mouth is not a functional way to breathe at all. This is one perfect example of how the respiratory dysfunction strains the cardiovascular, musculoskeletal and neurological system. Inhaling through the nose creates dilation where as inhaling through the mouth creates constriction.

• **CO_2 is the primary factor for your breathing rate to increase or decrease and instructs the blood what to do with O_2.** There are receptors (chemoreceptors) in the veins and arteries that send information to the brain about CO_2 levels in the blood. As CO_2 levels rise, it releases stored O_2 from hemoglobin in the blood and travels to cells and muscles that need it. But when CO_2 is low, O_2 is not released from hemoglobin, the blood, because it is not needed. CO_2 is the main factor that releases O_2 at rest and during exercise. For this reason, CO_2 is a signal calling for O_2, showing work was produced and more O_2 is required. The blood does not give up O_2 as freely as you think. Your blood holds O_2 until it really needs to release it, until there is an affinity, an attraction, a need for it, from metabolic cellular reactions at rest to exercise when CO_2 levels rise rapidly because of working muscles and cells. It is a survival mechanism for the body. But like I just said, breathing through the mouth makes this process dysfunctional because of **poor breathing mechanics**.

• **CO_2 is more easily released from the body than O_2 perfusion.** O_2 needs the proper conditions to enter the capillary. CO_2 is a byproduct of cellular metabolism that is released from the body naturally. It has a higher and quicker rate of release because it does not require anything for it to be released, just exhaling. No attraction, no affinity is needed. We simply create breathing issues by breathing through our mouth, creating constantly low CO_2 levels. If the same were true for O_2 to be used and taken in so easily, we would be highly oxygenated people with high VO_2 levels, volume of oxygen. But unfortunately, it's not the same. Your mouth is just a secondary emergency way to breathe and used to eat. Controlling CO_2 through how we breathe is the key to O_2 utilization.

• **The body maintains a certain level of O_2 and CO_2 in the alveoli (100mm/hg O_2) (40 mm/hg CO_2) during a resting state.** The objective of nasal diaphragmatic breathing at rest is to produce the proper **exchanges** of O_2 and CO_2, to sustain the level needed to be functional and healthy. Therefore, breathing less per minute makes the heart more efficient to beat less per minute because of **more exchanges** in the lower lungs area. On the contrary, breathing through the mouth makes the lungs work harder increasing the breathing rate (hyperventilating) and directly increasing the heart rate per minute because of **fewer exchanges**. The heart has to pump harder and more, increasing the rate per minute because of O_2 deprivation to the heart and muscles, etc. It's not about clearing all your CO_2 because you need it! How you breathe is the difference between health and disease, vitality and fatigue, feeling young or old.

• **As oxygen demands increase during exercise, we need to meet those demands.** For this reason, by taking deeper, longer and fewer inhalations through the nostrils, we can neutralize the demand for oxygen more effectively into the bigger more abundant spaces of the lower lungs, using the whole lungs, where more alveolar sacs are present, maximizing volume and performance without strain. If you want this process to really be effective, increase the amount of capillaries and mitochondria's in your muscles as well, exactly what exercise does. This will make your body much more effective at utilizing O_2 during exercise and in a resting state.

• **Society has been misled into thinking that CO_2 is toxic and bad for you, when it is actually the opposite.** CO_2 is an important gas because it is a natural vasodilator. In the nasal passages there is a gas called nitric oxide (NO) that is produced naturally. In an abstract according to PubMed.gov, *Nitric oxide and the Paranasal Sinuses*, nitric oxide produces vasodilation, a natural dilating gas that expands the bronchial tubes and bronchioles, making it easier for more air to pass, delivering oxygen to the blood. NO also acts as an antimicrobial that filters the air in your nose preventing bacteria and pollutants from entering your body. Breathing through the nose keeps the presence of CO_2 in the airflow, at a minimal level, to maintain dilation. This is one significant quality that can only be achieved from nasal breathing and can solve many physical ailments by retraining the breathing process.

• **Vasodilation means that veins and arteries expand, stay open, which is what CO_2 promotes, not constriction.** This means the arteries and veins dilate for O_2 to be released in the areas of **high CO_2 concentrations**, where it is needed most. CO_2 relaxes muscles, stimulates nerves, especially to the brain, and reduces inflammation in joints and the body because of its dilation qualities. When CO_2 is produced, it signals and prepares the path for O_2. For example, when **CO_2 is high**, O_2 will be released from the blood easily to balance an acidic environment of CO_2 where CO_2 facilitates the process of vasodilation for O_2 delivery. When **CO_2 is low**, blood vessels constrict (vasoconstriction) and less O_2 is released (Bhor Effect) because there is no affinity (attraction) or need for it. If **CO_2 is low**, vasoconstriction affects the brain, organs, muscles, arteries, veins and the systemic. Vasoconstriction produces strain on the lungs, heart, arteries and veins affecting the function, integration and dynamics of the respiratory and cardiovascular systems. That is the beauty of CO_2's power, having the affinity to prepare and attract O_2. What depends on the success to maintain the ability to intake and release O_2 properly is based on CO_2 levels. This is especially important to sustain energy, health and vitality. It is extremely important for sports performance to keep veins and arteries under vasodilation to maintain energy and power.

Example: Make sure you are sitting down. Read first so you will understand the effects. Inhale and exhale through your mouth 5 to 8 times deeply. Wait for about one minute and you will start to feel lightheaded from mouth breathing within that minute. Relax for a few minutes reset and come back to focus. Now, perform the same number of repetitions keeping the mouth closed and only breathing through the nose 5 to 8 times the same way. You will notice the nose has more control over the flow of air than the mouth. The flow of air through the mouth is erratic and too much, that leads too expelling too much CO_2. The reason you felt lightheaded from mouth breathing is because the mouth expels too much CO_2 at one time. The nose provides regulation. When CO_2

levels fall, O_2 stays bounded and not released by the blood producing an alkaline state in the blood that constricts veins and arteries leading to lightheadedness. You may have felt a little lightheaded from the nasal breathing, but not as much or as high in comparison to mouth breathing, because your breathing is not trained.

UNCONSCIOUS EFFECTS OF POOR BREATHING MECHANICS

Many situations in life can change how we breathe from the nose to mouth from deep to shallow; like being sick with fever, flu, stress, depression, fear, sitting too much, fatigue, not sleeping well, being sedentary or from living the modern lifestyle. At some point poor breathing dynamics take over to imbalance life, physical health, create joint inflammation, increase blood pressure, and produce muscle pain and tension. We allow it to happen and train it into our system to adapt and function with it in everyday life. The problems that arise from breathing through your mouth and shallow breathing are: asthma, headaches, tight muscles (especially in the neck and back), inflexibility, fatigue, decreased cardiovascular capacity, increased heart rate, increased blood pressure, lung infections etc. On the contrary, there are many very important and crucial qualities that can be attained from breathing through the nose and not the mouth that can prevent the problems associated above.

Over time, it is the cardiovascular issues like increased heart rate and blood pressure that eventually become cardiovascular diseases, trickling down, producing other imbalances, diseases and disorders in the body. There's no buffer or control from breathing to establish the balance and function of pressure, tension and exchanges, so force and strain make the heart work harder. Doctors do not teach you how to breathe. They inspire and recommend you to exercise. It's up to you to make the unconscious breathing pattern conscious by using it. As you can see, breathing affects the respiratory system that affects the cardiovascular system's responses, impacting the musculoskeletal and central nervous system. Such is the power of breathing and all the unconscious systems' connections. Changing how you breathe will change how you feel and how you move. It will bring benefit and reward instantly because your breathing can adapt and adjust in an instant. You have the power to make the unconscious conscious.

You now know understand the power and capacity to change your life and health. Breath is your life force. It's your power. Its power is based on simplicity. You already breathe—inhale and exhale. The only adjustment you need is to breathe through the nose and train your breath. The challenge is not to fall into the bad habit of mouth breathing. Stay mindful of your breath and keep stress and emotions in check. What you are mindful of will start to construct your life. This is the reason you need to be aware of breathing, alignment and the things you eat and do in the moment, because they are going to construct your future habits and health. *Being mindful of your breath gives you control and power over your life.* Awareness and consciousness of the breathing pattern is a must. Losing awareness of the breathing pattern compensates instantly. Remember, it is an automatic function with a failsafe switch. Be conscious to breathe to produce the circuitry for health and exercise. Mindfulness is the key.

BREATHING IN MOVEMENT

When you know you are going to exert force to jump, sprint, tackle, push or pull, you generate pressure through breathing to be released into the exertion of the movement or to stabilize the movement. It all depends on the movement you are performing. The idea is to maintain abdominal tension naturally, as you breathe. Breathing in movement is like stretching a rubber band then letting it go to release it's energy. Remember, *"Inhalation encourages the contraction of most muscles and exhalation encourages their relaxation."* (Travell and Simons). Since the body can move and exert force in many different directions, breathing and exertion depends on the movement and direction. If you don't have pressure and tension then you won't generate force and power. Dr. Stuart

McGill refers to this as *"bracing breath"* He says, *"bracing breath transfers to the spine and muscles throughout the body."* The more intra-abdominal pressure produced from nasal diaphragmatic breathing, the more tension the abdominals and the core will have that can be transferred through movement: pressing, throwing, kicking, punching, jumping, running, etc. It is the reason why breathing transfers strength through and to muscles. Mouth breathers cannot do this effectively. They don't have a regulated breathing pattern that is functional or progressive. Mouth breathing does not produce the intra-abdominal pressure needed to produce abdominal tension nor has maximal inhalation power to be released in movement. Because of the lack of intra-abdominal pressure produced from mouth breathing, it does not produce abdominal and core stability effectively, an important reason why the spine develops poor posture and flexion (rounded spine), from the lack of stability.

When I teach clients to breathe, I teach them a few different ways to breathe during movement. One way is inhaling and exhaling through the nose. The second way is inhaling through the nose and exhaling through pursed lips. The second way of breathing releases CO_2 at a regulated rate and not too much so quickly, like open mouth breathing does. When you exhale using pursed lips, it is like blowing through a straw. There is a reflex in the exhalation of air through pursed lips that makes the abdominals tense and the core stabilize. Try it! Inhale through your nose for 3-5 seconds and exhale pushing the air through pursed lips, like blowing through a straw. The harder you push the air through pursed lips, the more the abdominals produce isometric contraction. I have taught this method to many students, clients and athletes because it is extremely beneficial to use during sports, strength training and running to maximize performance, power and energy. It is a very multi-useful and powerful way to breathe. Increasing the power of your breathing enhances core and abdominal tension. Enhancing the core and abdominal tension augments strength. Breathing properly maximizes and conserves energy. Many understand the reasons for their fatigue now, having to push and force through their exercises in the past. However, it is unnecessary to force exercise and strength if you are breathing correctly in your training, sustaining the needs for oxygen, pressure and tension to move. If you feel tired, check how you are breathing. Breathing needs to be normal and regular not forced and compensated. Your breath works with alignment and movement in an integrated and coordinated process, especially with stability. The joints and spine have a kinetic link and an unconscious neuromuscular connection to breathing. How you breathe influences posture and joint alignment.

The breathing techniques in this book will help you develop a functional breathing pattern that institutes good health and creates a stable core to transfer through mobility and movement. Sometimes it's a pace like when running and sometimes it's for more tension to move deeper into a strength pattern or to resolve movement. By breathing deeper and creating more core tension and stability, you can move more weight as well. Knowing, training and practicing breathing will put you on top of the competition. I have taught many people, including athletes, to dramatically improve their movements and sport. In rugby, I taught and trained players how to develop pressure and tension through breathing, coordinating it with their playing techniques to move the ruck, tackle and sprint. In judo, I taught and trained players how to throw more powerfully. For rowers, I taught them how to create a powerful endurance tank of energy. I have taught clients to breathe better from the improvement of posture to the development of the core. It is not necessary to learn yoga to improve your breathing. Yoga is a form of exercise that works with breathing. All forms of exercise should work with breathing first, alignment and stability second and movement third. It is the integration of the three that creates motion, functional efficiency and work as a catalyst setting the platform for a movement pattern and it's power: to throw, ruck, squat or lunge, etc. If you're not breathing correctly, you're not going to produce stability in the core and the pressure needed to produce tension for the abdominals, especially if you breathe into the chest. You cannot create and manipulate the core as a fulcrum to stabilize the spine and move powerfully. If you are not stable, then balance, coordination and transference of movement is difficult. Imagine jumping off a dock into the water. Now, imagine jumping into the water off a canoe. There is a big power difference between the two due to the stability of the platform in which you jump to coordinate the power to move. Breathing is the timing chain to coordinate and synchronize all functions in movement patterns, exercises and poses.

When you perform movement patterns and poses, think about how your breathing can best establish pressure for abdominal tension to transfer through the pattern or pose. This is essential when increasing the intensity of a movement or adding weight. The breath needs to be trained into movement through repetition, building the strength of the diaphragm to contract and relax, to be resilient. It matters how you breathe to the core in movement, not how much weight you can move physically. That comes later.

When I work on breathing with someone, I always ask: What sensations do you now feel? The answer I always get is, "I feel light and more upright." When posture is strong and balanced, you feel less tension and less gravity pulling on you, thus making you feel lighter and more energetic in your body, balancing energy. Alignment and stability thus communicates harmony to joints and muscles; preventing misalignment and instability from making adjustments in the body that use so much energy to maintain imbalance. How we respond to gravity's pull is what forms our proprioception system. Before you learn the breathing exercises find out if you are a chest or abdominal breather.

Chest or Abdominal Breathing Test

- Lie down on your back. Place your hands on your chest and abdomen.
- Start to breathe.
- Feel which rise's first—the chest or abdominals.

It is desirable to have the abdominals react and rise first to fill the bottom of the lungs and have air travel up to the chest. Breathing into the chest cannot pull air down into the bottom of the lungs. You are therefore not utilizing full capacity of the lungs because you are not using your diaphragm. A quick correction is to lie on your stomach and clasp your fingers together. Place your forehead on the clasped fingers and breathe into the stomach through your nose. The floor will give pressure to the abdominals, providing stimulation to the diaphragm. Crocodile breathing is a good way to correct and learn how to breathe into the abdomen. It's also very relaxing.

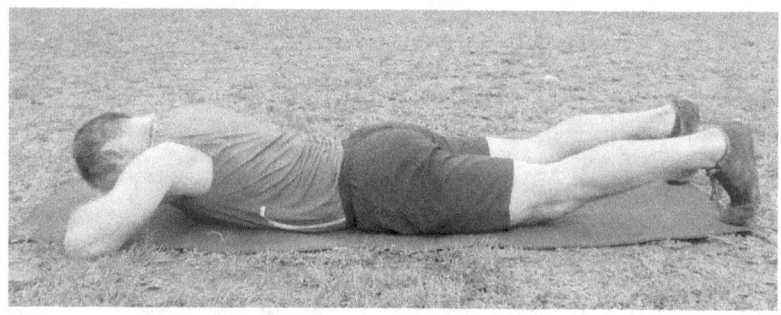

Another correction is to clasp your fingers together and place them on your stomach over your navel in a seated or standing position. Breathe in through your nose and place pressure on the abdominals by pushing the clasped hands into the abdominals as you inhale. As you push the hands on the abdominals, they will create tension. Use the breath to provide pressure as a foundation behind the abdominals. At the same time, pull your elbows into the ribcage. You will feel the lats and back muscles contract along with the abdominal tension and the inhalation.

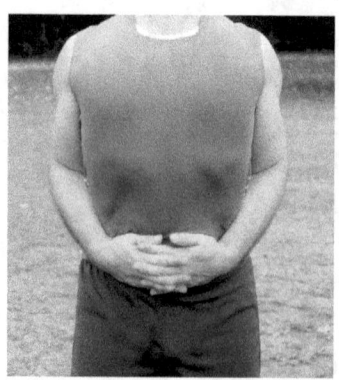

USING THE DIAPHRAGM FOR
RUNNING AND TRAINING

Many people begin their fitness program by jumping on a cardiovascular machine, watching TV and running like robots. They use machines to produce muscular strength without using their breath in any way integrated to movement. Being attuned to how the body moves and feels is important, but it requires awareness. Being mindful of your breathing during exercise, you can take its cues to help you regulate heart rate, be more efficient and more effective. Learning to breathe through the nose prevents the hearts beats per minute from spiking too high that can extend endurance. When strength training, it connects us to the nervous and musculoskeletal system to maximize strength production. Breathing can be trained and controlled to make changes in an instant.

During an exercise like running (when tension builds) it is preferable to control breathing—to establish pace, rhythm and take fewer deeper and longer breaths using the diaphragm, not more. Using nasal diaphragmatic breathing during running is more suitable for energy conservation as well. You need to take cues on when to inhale and exhale to train and regulate your breathing pattern. In the beginning, you will probably find your breathing rhythm is a bit erratic. Just keep focusing on inhaling through the nose and relaxing your breathing. You can also run by inhaling through the nose and exhaling through pursed lips to prevent the release of too much CO_2 and to maintain abdominal pressure. As you train your running, you will notice your breathing starts to get deeper and longer and will find slight pauses in your breathing, taking less breaths per minute and becoming more relaxed. More relaxed means the respiratory system is not straining and is performing functionally, efficiently and effectively. Nasal diaphragmatic breathing promotes relaxation of the nervous system and synchronizes the respiratory and cardiovascular systems performance optimally. Once you have established the rhythm and control of your breathing, you can synchronize the breathing with your foot strike. This is where you will economize and conserve energy more efficiently. But you need the breathing foundation first.

When running, **the inhalation** produces the contraction of the diaphragm to increase the volume of oxygen and stabilize the core and all the postural muscles to keep the torso stable and aligned to transfer forces. In the same breath, it facilitates and supports muscular contractions that maintain joint alignment, stability and movement strength overall through your foot strike. Therefore, inhalation activates the diaphragm that produces the pressure for the core and tension for the abdominals, to stabilize the forces generated through the foot strike. The secret to breathing and running is to inhale longer and deeper through the nose using the diaphragm. This helps to maintain pressure and stability in the core and you will have the greatest amount of stability and optimal joint alignment at the time of impact, not less, to propel you forward with the spring in your step to run effortlessly. Remember, there is more power jumping off the dock, the stable platform, than the canoe, the unbalanced platform, to propel you forward. You always need to have pressure to maintain stability and tension transference.

When you run, for example, try inhaling through your nose for 6 running steps or 4 seconds and then exhale through your nose for 3 running steps or 2 seconds. Continue this technique through your running. You can always adjust the ratio for yourself personally. It is more about what gives you the most control in the beginning and expanding upon that foundation for progression. You don't have to be stuck to the numbers the whole time. You have to train the process. You have to listen to what the body needs at the time of performance. Your breathing will tell you what it needs to do, if you are mindful to it. Your breathing rate may not be the same all the time. Sometimes you breathe deeper and longer; and minutes later shorter and faster through the nose. It all depends on many factors from nutrition, to having a clear mind, to rest and recovery. Learn to adjust your running around your breathing. If you need to run slower, run slower and train the natural functional breathing process to maintain proper functional breathing as a good habit. If you don't, you will compensate progression that will lead to strain, decreasing your running time and power. Train utilizing the lower lung to develop a higher volume of oxygen, in turn, running will develop capillaries and mitochondria that also improve the efficiency and effectiveness of oxygen utilization. Not listening can lead you down a different path creating fatigue because you are trying to do more than the system can handle at that time.

In strength training, you need to control and train your breathing to produce more stability through repetitions. You need to activate the core through the inhalation of the nose to produce a high stabilizing pressure needed through movement because of adding weights and load. The high stabilizing pressure makes you stronger instantly because it stimulates the nervous and neuromuscular system's amplitude and electrical frequency. When you increase pressure, you increase tension and that is what stimulates the nervous system's circuitry to transmit power through the musculoskeletal system to perform. When you exhale, you exhale through pursed lips and that activates the reflex for the abdominals to stabilize that facilitates the spine's stability. How you breathe is important in repetition for timing, coordination and synchronization. Most people develop subpar strength and potential because they only train the musculoskeletal system not the respiratory or nervous system integration properly. The nervous system is what produces the strength and power for the musculoskeletal system. But like anything, you need to practice and use the proper programing to facilitate the best results. When you stop practicing breathing techniques you lose power, much like when you stop strength training, you lose some strength. It needs to be a daily practice.

As you perform strength programs or running with poor breathing mechanics, the loss of stability gets transferred to the joints through motion. Losing stability is like losing the shock absorbers on your car. They can't diffuse and transfer the forces applied and generated to and through the whole body. Instead, force gets stuck and absorbed by the joints and muscles individually, producing pain or strain. As you continue to train with poor breathing technique, you are transferring and training the compensations and inefficiency through the system. Training the process of nasal diaphragmatic breathing is important because each process triggers the next. Inhaling through the nose triggers the diaphragm to pull down the bottom of the lungs to increase the space and capacity for more oxygen volume. At the same time, the inhalation produces the pressure and stability for the core and spine, triggering the nervous systems power. Without using the breath as the trigger, the integration of the cardiovascular, nervous and musculoskeletal system will lead to less effective results. Without inhaling through the nose first, the sequence will be compensated. I have observed notable improvements in clients' strength, range of motion and mobility, as well as the resolution of strain and pain, as they learn how breathing and stability work together. Nasal diaphragmatic breathing is therefore the missing piece to complete the puzzle for increased performance, fitness, vitality and health.

Nasal Breathing	Mouth Breathing
Learned as a baby.	Learned as an adult.
Longer, deeper breaths, lower breathing rate.	Shorter, quicker, erratic faster breathing rate.
Lower heart rate and blood pressure.	Higher heart rate and blood pressure.
Uses the diaphragm.	Does not use diaphragm.
Breathes into the lower lungs where there are vast amounts of exchanges increasing volume of oxygen.	Breathes into the upper lungs for minimal amount of exchanges decreasing the volume of oxygen.
Produces pressure to strengthen the core, abdominals and the spines stability.	Cannot do.
Uses Nitric Oxide.	Cannot do.
Balances O2 and CO2 exchange.	Offsets the balance.
Parasympathetic (Slow).	Sympathetic(Rapid and Fast).

ONE-MINUTE BREATHING TEST

WARNING: If you find any of the breathing exercises difficult and challenging, never hold your breath unless you have been trained to do so first. You have to learn to adapt and adjust to the exchange of O_2 and CO_2 as well as the pressure. Holding your breath is detrimental if you are not trained to do so and have respiratory or cardiovascular issues.

Let's see how many breaths you take in one minute. Just breathe normally for one minute. Use your everyday breath, that is, don't inhale so your shoulders rise and struggle to get the last bit of air in to perform fewer breaths in the time. If you are a mouth breather then breathe through your mouth. If you breathe rapidly, then do it for the test or you will be missing the point here. If you don't know what is dysfunctional, you will not know how to advance.

- One breath is both an inhalation and an exhalation.
- Breathe how you breathe normally.

Remember this is practice and training. It does not mean you have to walk around trying to breathe for three breaths a minute normally, like in your practice. Before you begin, take your heart rate for one minute and your blood pressure, if you have the capability. Chart your progress using breaths per minute and heart rate. Retest after every three to five faithful practice days.

Breaths in one minute, the results from the one-minute test:
    Excellent: 3 breaths or less per minute
    Good: 3 - 12 breaths per minute
    Average/ Normal: 12 - 18 breaths per minute
    Poor: 18 or more breaths per minute

I take two and a half to three breaths a minute in my **breathing practice, my training.** My resting heart rate is 48. My first breath is 22 seconds, the second is 25, and I start the third breath at 47 seconds. When I breathe **normally at rest** for the one-minute test, I breathe about 6 breaths per minute. The test is not the training. I test for six breaths with normal breathing in one minute without focusing on trying to inhale deeper and exhale slower. I train and practice using two and a half to three breaths per minute, concentrating on control to relax, slowly inhaling deeply and slowly exhaling to create capacity, volume, strength and pressure. I do this for about 5-8 minutes of time to strength train the breathing pattern. I also focus on it for many minutes spaced throughout the day. The breathing practice, the training, helps my breaths per minute become lower at rest. When time gets longer for breathing, it is good. It is becoming more efficient.

Pulse/Heart Rate (min)	Breathing Rate (min)	CO_2 % In the Alveoli
Excellent 48	3	7.5
Good 50	4	7.4
Good 52	5	7.3
Good 55	6	7.1
Good 57	7	6.8
Good 60	8	6.5
Good 65	10	6.0
Good 70	12	5.5
Average 75	15	5.0
Poor 80	20	4.5
Poor 90	26	4.0
Poor 100	30	3.5

This chart is just a piece of the full chart, The Buteyko Table of Health Zones, created by Dr. Buteyko. This piece shows the pulse rate, breathing rate and CO_2 levels for health and disease based on nasal breathers being excellent and mouth breathers being poor. Also note that, CO_2 is higher with a lower heart rate and breathing rate.

As you become trained, you don't need to breathe as much and your breath will take pauses before the next breath through the nose. Try it. Sit down. Take a deep breath through the nose at pace, not too fast, can be slow. Now, exhale out fully through the nose. Now notice when you needed to take the next breath? It was not instantly. Therefore, you are not breathing in and out constantly because the body does not require another breath just yet, especially at rest. This is the effect of nasal diaphragmatic breathing; using more surface area in the lungs effectively for more O_2 and CO_2 exchanges with less breaths, not more breaths, maintaining the balance. Nasal diaphragmatic breathing produces a stronger and higher-pressure gradient than the mouth that affects the control, inhalation and exhalation. Like I said before, you can inhale and exhale more air breathing through your mouth, but it is not functional and has less control. Mouth breathing is **not hardwired** to utilize and regulate O_2 and CO_2 properly. You are using less surface area; breathing into the top of the lungs with too much airflow and strain that cannot perform the exchanges functionally.

It has been proven that most people who are mouth breathers breathe more than 12 times a minute and may suffer from COPD, asthma or allergies. It has been scientifically proven that heart disease is linked to shortness of breath and oxygen deprivation to the heart from mouth breathing. Breathing through the mouth has a high correlation to high blood pressure. It also has a high link with anxiety, depression, stress, tension and many emotional disorders. Dr. Buteyko, a Russian physician, found that all sick people who have asthma, bronchitis, heart disease, diabetes, cancer, etc., have accelerated respiratory breathing patterns. Having an increased breathing pattern and rate means carbon dioxide is deficient, making oxygen delivery to the cells low and the natural pause in the breathing pattern is missing. On the contrary, Dr. Buteyko showed that controlling your breathing regulates the cardiovascular, immune, nervous, and digestive system of the body.

Chapter 2
Breathing Development, Techniques and Practice
"The most perfect technique is that which is not noticed at all." -Pablo Casals

THE BREATHING EXERCISES: ACTIVATING THE DIAPHRAGM

When most people exercise, run or perform strength training, one of the reasons for their fatigue is because they are not breathing properly. This impacts the integration between the systems, affecting endurance, strength, power output and results.

There are many different ways to breathe. The two types I focus on work with nasal diaphragmatic breathing. The first is breathing in and out of the nose that is required for more repetitive aerobic type of movements like running. The second type of breathing is breathing in through the nose and hissing the air out the mouth with pursed lips. The second type of breathing is used for movement patterns and strength training because you need to maintain pressure in the core when moving weights around, stretching muscles and moving joints in different angles and directions to maintain stability. Exhaling through pursed lips does this perfectly. Bracing breath (pursed lips) maintains a higher level of power and stability. The hiss out of the mouth (pursed lips) activates abdominal stability, maintaining high pressure for the exhalation and exertion of the movement being executed. Combining both gives you a powerful combination in sports like rugby, hockey, martial arts, MMA, judo, football, etc. The hiss is also effective when running, especially for speed. What's most important is that you inhale through the nose and exhale your air through minimal space, like the nose or pursed lips, to retain air and pressure. All in all, it depends on what is more comfortable for you. How fast you release the exhalation is what makes the difference: pausing or slightly holding depends on the activity and sport at hand. As you develop this breathing technique, the abdominals, diaphragm and lungs become stronger; as well as your stability and power to move.

Making Contact with the Diaphragm – Learning to Inhale

- Sit up straight or stand. Try to keep the shoulders back. The shoulders will create tension on the spine's postural alignment producing connectivity for the abdominals to react.
- Breathe in through your nose.
- As you breathe in, keep the abdominals tight to prevent the stomach from distending. **You will feel the tension in the abdominals, ribcage and up the spine when you don't push the stomach out.** This technique will strengthen your lungs, the diaphragm, the abdominals, the core and postural muscles, producing stability between the abdominals and spine all at the same time. You are not sucking in your stomach. You are tensing and creating a wall in the abdominals that tightens from the inhalation.
- Create pressure as far as you are comfortable. Keep the abdominals tight producing a wall of tension matching the breath's pressure coming in.
- Exhale at any pace you want for now through the nose or pursed lips. Just concentrate on inhaling, producing pressure for the abdominals to create a wall of tension for a strong diaphragmatic contraction. Let the abdominals and breath go, and feel the breath naturally exhale.
- Practice for 10 breaths.
- If you are having an issue tightening the abdominals, use a belt. Don't make the belt extremely tight, because when you inhale, the abdominals will tighten. Make the belt tight enough where you can slide one finger between the belt and your stomach and then do the inhalations.

35

Bracing the abdominals with the inhale starts to develop the core. If you distend your stomach when you inhale, you will not feel the pressure and tension in the core, spine and the rib cage. If you have a rounded spine, slouched and rounded shoulders, try to sit up straight with good posture and pull the shoulders back as you do the breathing exercises. This will help contract the muscles conducive for alignment. Go slow. When your posture is poor the diaphragm and other muscles in that area are probably restricted.

(Note: Many programs practice stomach distention, but such a practice lacks the ability to transfer tension. Sucking the abdominals in makes the spine round.)

The Hiss: Learning to Exhale

- Breathe in through the nose to the abdominals with abdominal bracing tension.
- Keep your lips pursed.
- Now, instead of letting the breath and the abdominal tension go like the first technique, keep the abdominals tight and push the air through pursed lips. It should feel like blowing through a straw. As you do this, the abdominals will stay tight automatically from the reflex. (The more your mouth is open the less pressure and the less tension the abdominals produce with no reflex.) Let it happen naturally right now.
- You will feel a belt forming around the hips and lower back. As you hiss you will feel the pressure build up strengthening the lungs.
- Don't worry about breathing at full capacity here. Inhale for about 3 to 5 seconds. Tighten the abdominals around the inhalation. Then, exhale with pursed lips activating the abdominals isometric contraction. Practice for 10 breaths, inhaling and exhaling. Build up to long inhalations and exhalations to train the lungs.

Breath, stability and pressure create transference of tension and pressure through the body radiating strength and stability through the joints and muscles (musculoskeletal and neuromuscular systems), especially for strong movements. Practice this exercise regularly to strengthen your lungs and incorporate it into your life and your training programs. It will help to improve your health and performance in running or any other activity. Practice the inhalation and exhalation deeply using the natural pause after the inhalation and after the exhalation. Try to practice for a given amount of time. After you practice and return your breathing to a normal way, you will see instant results lowering your breaths per minute from about 30-50 % and your natural pauses get longer. You feel the effects instantly to reverse the detrimental affects immediately for health but you need to train to enhance those effects for more performance. Make it a habit for your lungs to be functional to regulate the body and maintain health.

The next exercises are breathing exercises to expand your functionality.

Lung Resiliency
Breathe in slowly and deeply. Exhale slowly to develop breathing capacity, strength, endurance and stamina.
- Stand or sit comfortably.
- As you breathe in through your nose, tighten your abdominals to match the breath you are slowly inhaling. The deeper you breathe, the tighter you want to make the abdominals. Feel like a balloon is filling up inside your stomach but your stomach is not distending.
- Try to breathe into the lower abdominal basin below your navel.
- As you tighten the abdominals more, you will feel the diaphragm tighten more pulling down.
- Keep the abdominals tight, so as you breathe, pressure and tension will cover a greater surface area. Practice slowly to learn

37

how to train and maintain this space and pressure.

- To strengthen your breathing, breathe in deeper and tighten the abdominals more to increase the power of the breath coming in. It is like hooking your two index fingers and trying to pull them apart, isometrically increasing the tension.
- Don't push out your stomach.
- Actively exhale by hissing the air out through pursed lips. Try to maintain control of the pressure when exhaling. Depending on how hard you push your air out and how tight the lips are, makes the abdominals tighten more or for less. So, it is a good abdominal exercise by just using your breath.
- Find the natural pause in between each breath and after the exhalation.
- Repeat 10 times.

If you breathe out of an open mouth, you will not maintain pressure or tension. If you need to breathe out of the mouth, then breathe. But resist the temptation to open your mouth. **Breathe if you need to and never force it!**

The Hiss Keeps the Abdominals Pressurized.
- An open mouth decreases abdominal pressure.
- A slightly open mouth trains you to retain pressure.
- A closed mouth holds pressure.

When running you may use softer pursed lips and during strength use a tighter pursed lip to produce more pressure.

Stamina – Ladder Breaths
You can start breathing in for a count of 5 seconds and then exhale for a count of 5 seconds, then 6 and 6, 7 and 7, 8 and 8, 9 and 9, 10 and 10. Then, work your way back down to 5. Choose a time that is

comfortable for you. Try to do it for 3 to 5 minutes. It is easy to do just a few times. You need to build up the strength of your breathing for stamina and endurance over time. You can also breathe in for 5 seconds and breathe out slowly for 8 seconds. Always try to do it for a given amount of incremental time. Your breath will get stronger and you will be learning control.

CAUTION: Do not strain or force breathing. Stop if it feels uncomfortable. If you have issues with your lungs and heart, seek your doctor's advice first before proceeding with the exercises.

Inhaling slowly will exercise the diaphragm's contraction, increase the capacity of VO_2 and develop the lungs' pressure system. Slowly exhaling will eccentrically strengthen the diaphragm and train the lung's pressure system, developing endurance and resiliency. You can develop more strength on the eccentric contraction (exhalation) in your breath training, just like in your muscular strength training. Similarly to muscles, you want the lungs to be resilient as well. You ultimately want to train your lungs to take fewer breaths per minute at rest, during exercise, running and training by increasing the length of your breath to increase VO_2 and core stability at the same time. Such efficiency leads to highly effective conditioning. You have to imagine that the heart rate, blood pressure and breathing rate are gauges for the body. If breathing is not efficient, when it is belabored, the gauges will adjust for those responses.

Use control and direction of your breath when breathing. Believe it or not, just because you breathe does not mean you breathe evenly to the core. People breathe more into one side than the other, which develops breathing asymmetry and core strength imbalance. This imbalance affects the stability of the abdominals and projects spinal misalignments, shoulder issues, neck issues and poor posture, resulting in structural asymmetry. When structural asymmetry is present, it leads to dysfunctional movement. To feel for asymmetries, as you breathe, use your fingers to press into the right and left sides of the abdominals. You will feel a spot a litter softer than the rest of the abdominal area. When you find the softer spot, press your fingers into the spot and breathe into your fingers pressure at the same time and feel the abdominals tighten like the other spots. The breath aligns the spine from the sacrum and lumbar all the way up to the neck and the base of the skull.

Breathing is the catalyst activating synergy to synchronize movement. Perform slowly to produce a well-prepared, strong, coordinated foundation that can handle increases of force, speed and intensity for progression. It all starts with breathing. Breathing and movement are about improving quality first, not quantity. Quantity will build from practicing quality. But quality will not build from just practicing quantity. Development is what you put in to reap prevention, benefit and reward. More is not better until you are functionally efficient and trained. Know this in strength training as well. Feeling tired from the breathing exercises is a sign that you need to rethink how you perform fitness, strength and conditioning programing, even how you live life. You must consciously, consistently, competently practice to make it a habit. At any point go back and see if your breaths per minute lowered. If you get quick results, great! If not, trust that practice hacks away the barriers and years of dysfunction and inefficiency.

I always feel stronger after my breathing practice. It is the reason I get stronger in my second, third and fourth sets with strength and movement. The strength of the breath gets deeper and generates more power in the neuromuscular and nervous system. Strength and performance progression relies on increased pressure, tension and stability. Breathing supersedes movement in developing strength. Therefore, strength increases in sets and you can maintain power in performance if you know how to use your breath in recovery and activity. You should be getting stronger in your sets, not weaker. This has much to do with the strength, stamina and endurance of your breathing to move loads in strength training and/or running.

The students I work with cannot believe how fast they start to move and how strong they become in one or two sessions. For example, a client I had in the past would press a weight 4 times the first set, 5 times the second set and 6 times the third set. Not bad for one session. But they all say the same thing—they realized they had been breathing in totally the wrong manner, which affected how they performed athletically and strength and cardiovascular exercise. They would say that the lack of endurance and strength in their breathing made them weaker and more tired. So, their strength decreased. Maintaining breathing, pressure and tension over time causes strength to increase, not decrease, until fatigue sets-in. The beautiful thing about breathing is, you can do it anytime, any day and anywhere. It works quickly. The hard part is, making it habitual.

Chapter 3
Stability- The Platform For Mobility and Movement

"If you don't have stability and alignment you will not have optimal range of motion, flexibility or effective movement to produce strength or power." - Jason Kelly

THE CORE IS NOT JUST ABS

By this time you know what the core is and how it works from performing the breathing techniques. You now feel that breathing through your nose activates the diaphragm. You now understand that breathing is the primary mechanical component that is responsible for the respiratory, cardiovascular, musculoskeletal and nervous systems functional integration.

On the physical level, if you draw a circle around the navel, the hips and the lower back, anything in this area directly affects and develops the core. Breathing, the abdominals, hips and spine comprise the core's functional pieces. Developing and progressing the core's strength is dependent on the functional pieces positions, stability and alignment to establish its power source. The stronger the core, the more power you can produce, transfer, coordinate, synchronize and ramify through training, performance or daily movements. When you think about strength and power you should think about breathing and alignment to activate and power the core. Synchronization is the key and needs to be included into your movement training, not just isolated muscle contractions.

Training the core requires you to train it in all movements, not in isolation like crunches'. The core is not isolated nor is it just abdominal muscular contractions, as society tends to think. People love doing crunches without having any knowledge about their ramifications.

- Crunches are detrimental, creating a strong abdomen but also wreaking havoc on the spine at rest, pulling it forward into a rounded posture.
- Crunches produce isolated strength that ramifies imbalance and weakness to other joints and muscles, disrupting the center of gravity. This imbalance renders the core ineffective because you are strengthening one muscle without the other in your motion.
- When you don't move from the core, your center of gravity, you produce joint misalignment and compensations in mobility and motion that imbalance strength (strength on one side produces weakness on the other like crunches; strong abdomen weak spine), decrease range of motion and mobility. Losing alignment of the spine limits and decreases your ability to perform other exercises effectively.
- This disruption of the core makes other joints of the body reconfigure their stability to support misalignment, creating limitations in movement. Joints shift based on what other joints are doing in the body. For example; crunches create a strong abdomen and produce spinal misalignment by rounding the spine that repositions the shoulders and neck forward into poor alignment, losing range of motion; from sitting too much the hips tilt back and causes the spine to round forward that affects the mobility and alignment of the shoulders and neck as well as your knees and ankles. This affects movement for the worst.
- When joints shift into misalignment, muscles become tense and lose flexibility and imbalance strength because they are maintaining an imbalanced and misaligned joint and structure because the joint is not doing it's job– stabilizing; hence the functional operating system becomes dysfunctional.
- In alignment, the muscles have balanced tension and strength that functions properly. Muscles contract to stabilize joints in alignment for other muscles to stretch and move.

What strengthens the core is everything working together, the synchronization, not one specific thing. Over strengthening or weakness in one aspect of the core unconsciously sabotages alignment and balance. The core produces strength through balance and leverage that travels through the whole body and is more advantageous than isolated muscular strength, such as crunches. Movements like crunches do not transfer into movement patterns, no matter if you are standing up, playing rugby, soccer, running, wrestling or judo, etc. Muscular strength isolation produced from crunches, threatens to undermine movement performance and range of motion in movements like plank, pushup, overhead presses, dead lift, etc., where spinal alignment is essential to elicit the proper results. Training crunches for abdominal isolation develops strength that will work against itself, in sports performance, fitness classes, running and strength and conditioning training.

Without core stability in a squat, the spine moves forward; in a push-up the lower back sags; in a lunge the spine flexes forward; lifting the arm up causes the spine to lean to the side or hyperextend. When you run with the spine flexed rounded forward, your joints, like the knees and neck, and your spine absorb more shear force causing pain and strain because of poor core stability and possibly poor hip stability. Looking at the issues more closely through the functional microscope, breathing and the core tend to be the hidden, buried issues. People move and train unconsciously without alignment and a fully developed core.

It is important to train the core as the center of gravity and build strength there from different movements. The foundation for this type of training is to expose the core to many different movements, training the core to be stronger at its primary functional position. Most people have it all wrong in strength training, only training the surface level of muscles: not including breathing, alignment and stability in their approach. Training the core and the body in many different positions, changing the center of gravity, develops better performance and increases strength because of practicing leverage. As a result, it makes the center—the core—reactive, stronger, more coordinated, educated and perceptive, understanding movement.

One very important reason I wrote this book was for you to realize that movement was the third factor in performing a movement pattern, pose or exercise. When you create a movement like a lunge, pushup or squat, these movements are just movements that create tension for you to strength train your breathing, alignment and core. Most people see it in reverse, training muscles as the primary result. If you can't breathe functionally, no matter how much weight you can move, it won't work well in the world of practical movement. Without core stability in movement, you produce inefficient and compensated movement and transfer it into other exercises. Shifting the center of gravity, the core, has a more profound effect on movement than piling on weights for strength, especially for performance. Most people cannot master simplicity to function first in their own movement patterns using their own body weight before proceeding to add weights to their movements. Strength and power is like a wild horse, it is something you need to know how to harness, tame and move, not just develop.

Personally, I've experienced the importance of the core—from all the years of strength training, physical conditioning, playing soccer for sixteen years, rugby for seventeen years, and from all the years of wrestling and judo. Remember, that breathing and the core are crucial for endurance and stamina in a sixty-minute training session, a ninety-minute game, through your day and daily tasks. In rugby, you need the power of the core to sustain being tackled, tackling, holding up your opponent and to drive a maul, meaning driving an opponent off the ball. If you are not familiar with the game of rugby, watch a game for a few minutes and you will begin to understand the importance of breathing and the core. In wrestling and judo the core gives you the necessary power you need through the arms and legs as leverage. When running, the core provides the necessary stability for the spine to maintain alignment when running.

Without breathing, the core will not be coordinated and you will not develop reactions and reflexes for speed and transitions properly.

You can move the biggest muscle guy with leverage and core power in rugby, judo or any sport. The stronger the core the more leverage you can produce through the body. The key to leverage is the fulcrum. By increasing the strength of breathing and the core, the fulcrum, the levers get stronger to move. If the fulcrum gets stronger, you can increase your strength training in short order. Learning to access the core will make the vital difference when progressing and evolving movement.

JOINT STABILITY

Joint stability is important in preserving joint alignment to maintain a functional, optimal and efficient position. Joint alignment dictates, controls and coordinates range of motion, muscle flexibility and mobility. By contracting muscles, you stabilize a joint's alignment, for example, the glutes and the hip joints. The glutes' strength and contraction keeps the hip joints in a stable aligned and balanced position when standing. It prevents the hip flexors from developing too much tension that pulls the hips forward into a tilt, decreasing range of motion and destabilizing the lumbar. Each joint has to shift as other joints shift whether it is for good or for bad. Maintaining the hip alignment allows the opposing muscles, like the quads, to have optimal flexibility and range of motion and to contract for other muscles like the hamstrings to stretch properly. With joints like the knee and ankle, they will move more efficiently and effectively from an aligned joint position. A stable, aligned joint produces the best mechanical advantages for range of motion, joint mobility and flexibility.

Joint compensation and misalignment, on the other hand, is an unconscious process. Sitting too much, developing poor posture and breathing through your mouth are just a few examples of how the body unconsciously shifts and moves into misalignment and loses stability. When these shifts happen, we are not mindful or aware of them because we don't feel them happen. But through time, we feel their effects and results, especially when strength training or running because you need alignment to distribute forces properly. Imbalance and misalignment

46

cannot do this well. Imagine driving a car with the axels bent. As you drive slowly, you will feel the car wobble up and down. Now, put some speed to it, the speed adds force that definitely will break the bent axel or damage another area or part of the car because the misalignment cannot handle the increase in speed and force.

Joint stability is one of the most important factors in functional movement. It allows motion to transfer. Joint stability is needed to move and direct energy joint to joint. Each step you take to walk, run, jump, lunge, squat, push or pull is based on the stability platform. In a squat, if you round your spine or lean it too far forward, your core is not stabilizing. Poor core stabilization affects the ankles and knees losing all the stability that the core and spine transfers from an erect position. Try it. Lunge with just a little bit of range of motion. You don't need much to feel this example. First, use a rounded spine and lunge three times as in photo 1. Now, pull your shoulders back or just lean back as in photo 2 and lunge three times. You should have felt a huge difference in transference of stability to the foot, ankle, knees and hips in the motion by just straightening your spine and pulling the shoulders back. You need stability and alignment to transfer forces properly through the body to create strength for the whole body, not isolated strength.

Photo 1

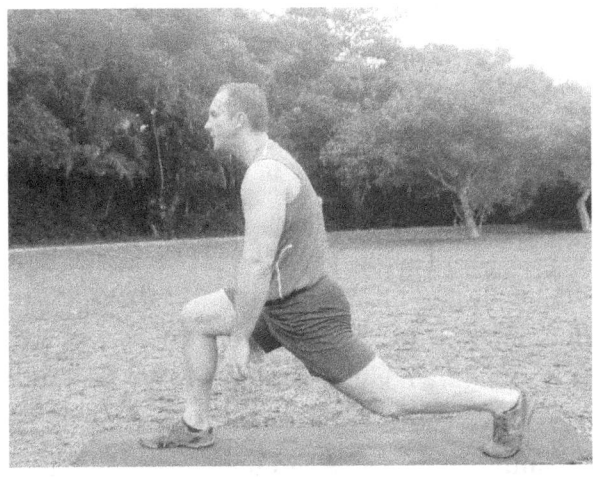

Photo 2

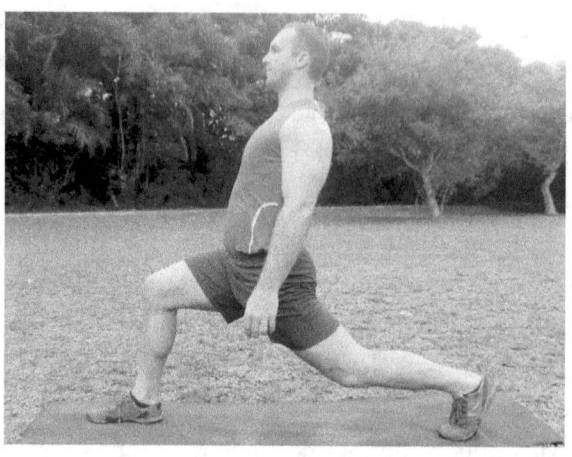

In photo one, the result is a lunge that moves but really does nothing for your body to strengthen breathing, the musculoskeletal, nervous and neuromuscular systems. What's more, in a shoulder press the lat (back muscles) and scapular muscles contract to stabilize the shoulder joint to press the weight and straighten your arm over your head. The lat contraction is absolutely necessary to stabilize and ground the shoulder joint for the arm to produce range of motion. If your spine is rounded forward, shoulder mobility is compensated and has less range to produce motion because of misalignment of the spine, as you can see in photo one above. As you keep loading shoulder mobility without stability and alignment of the spine, pain ensues, impingement develops and injury is lurking. Your movement is ineffective. Consequently, you begin to transfer ineffectiveness to other movements, developing pain and the beginning of bad movement habits. You start to function differently for many movement patterns.

In my training, I focus on stability and alignment, and to move that stability and alignment into ranges of motion. I don't try to justify range of motion without the functional foundation. I use my joints to move and let my muscles respond by contracting to stabilize the joints' position to allow range of motion and flexibility to be optimal. I don't focus on flexibility programing. It happens through my strength and movement training. Flexibility is the result. For example, in photos 3 and 4, performing a body weight dip, I breathe in to stabilize the abdominals and contract the lats and the back muscles to stabilize the scapulas. I contract the quads and glutes as well. This allows me to move into a deep range of motion with a straight spine. The same occurs with a push up. Breathing in to contract the abdominals and lats on the descent to the floor stabilizes the shoulder joint. This maintains alignment that allows more range of motion to stretch the chest. As you ascend in the dip and the pushup, keeping the lats contracted, maintains scapular and shoulder joint stability and balances strength development between the chest and the back.

Photo 3

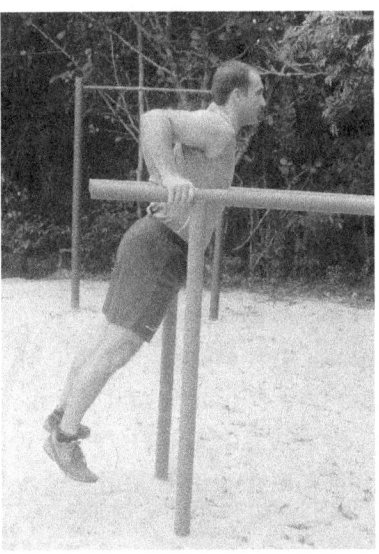

Photo 4

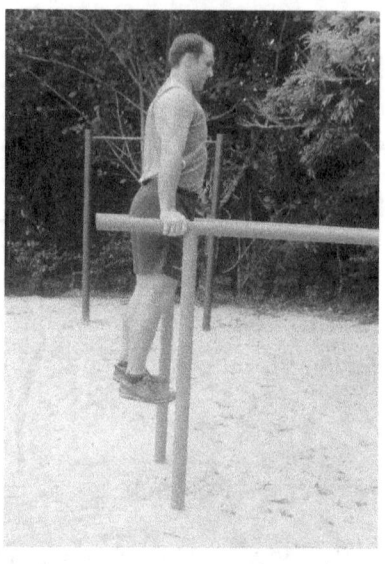

As my muscles stretch it's not just a passive stretch, it is a loaded controlled stretch through movement that augments strength. Similar to a cable holding up the span of a bridge, it is being stretched but maintaining it's tension, power, strength and alignment without being overstretched to maintain the forces applied. The more you stabilize a joint in a movement, pose or exercise, the more control and strength you have to move into range of motion effectively. All this teaches your body and joints how to maintain alignment and produce the linkage, leverage and synergy to move and strengthen the whole body. The nasal diaphragmatic breathing initiates this whole process. Don't think about speed right now. Speed comes when you have control of the movement and all the functional integrations (stability, mobility, contraction and flexibility) that produce range of motion working together. Society misses this valuable piece of strength development by focusing on strengthening specific muscles, speed and how much weight they can move with a poorly functioning body rather than strengthening the functional aspects for strength development and progression.

I see many people performing chest dips rounding the spine

forward as in photo 5. They are strengthening misalignment and losing the development of the linkage in muscular strength. Just because you can produce more range of motion by compensating the spine to round forward, does not mean it is productive, much like the lunge you just performed. You develop strength under instability and misalignment. People compensate joint stability for range of motion. Without the stability platform in movement, you will create force on a joint and imbalanced muscular strength that will produce strain, pain or injury. Stability creates the foundation for movement to function. The foundation's stability is going to be a critical factor to support the forces imposed on the body.

Photo 5

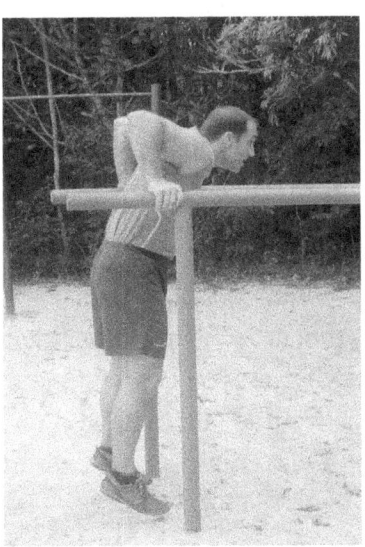

Chapter 4
Breathing and Movement and Sport Performance.
Don't lower your expectations to meet performance. Raise your level of performance to meet your expectations. –Ralph Marston

Depending on your movement depends on when to inhale and exhale. Sometimes it's quick and sometimes you hold and pause. The inhalation produces intra-abdominal pressure. When you produce a movement, you contract muscles during the inhalation phase that will increase your power on the exhalation. For example, when you punch, kick, throw or jump, etc., you inhale and load the movement creating pressure and tension and release it through the exhalation. The greater amount you can inhale, the stronger the core, the greater amount of pressure and tension you create, can be released as power through your movement. Depending on the sport depends on how to breathe, which I usually train individually for each sport as well as the athletic position.

Unfortunately, the mastery of breathing is pushed to the curb for the sake of strength training, performance and quantity. Your regimen should be about how your movements strengthen your breath and how your breath strengthens your movement, not just muscular strength. That is what you need to practice and take with you on the field, on the court, on the mat or in the ring. Think about exertion for movement and stabilization for a moment. To throw in judo, you need to breathe in as you are setting up the technique into the movement, to exhale at the throwing point. A rugby tackle or a defensive lineman in football, his strongest point is on the peak of inhalation as he hisses for exhalation. For a hockey player's slap shot, he breathes in on the wind up and exhales on the slap shot for power, likewise for a tennis swing or golf swing. What your sport or training is will define when to release the breath or when to breathe for power.

Each way you see it there is transference of power from breathing to the core through the movement. For this reason, you develop the core as a reactor. Then, learn to contract muscles with the core reactor, so like the recoil of the rubber band, you will have explosive power in your punch, kick, throw, swing, slap shot, jump, run, tackle, sprint, press or push, whatever the movement. As you train your breath in the movement, it becomes habitual and faster and you will not need to think about it. When you don't need to think about it, it becomes intuitive; and this is where speed and reflexes begin to enhance and evolve.

Train breathing into the movement slowly in the beginning to get all the muscles to contract and stretch appropriately with the inhalation and the core. Visualize the linkage of power coming from the breath and the core as you contract muscles to stabilize and move. Once you can visualize this blueprint mentally and do it slowly, then you can add speed. This will improve reflexes as well. The brain blueprints movement. It works on a feedback and a feed-forward mechanism. When you can do movements and perform slowly, you develop the breathing, stability and stamina to contract and stretch muscles to move while maintaining alignment. Alignment is important because it will provide maximal range of motion and the ability to create leverage (the ability to move a weight heavier than you can normally move) as well as the prevention of pain and injury because the body moves functionally and well. All this is done through your power of breathing. When you train fast before slow; you don't develop a functional system and can't perform this process. Train slowly and progress into speed. If you don't train it, you will not have this power, nor progress optimally.

The cerebellum may act as a feedback control system for slow movements and a feed forward controller for fast movements. (From University of Texas Health Science Center at Houston – http://neuroscience.uth.tmc.edu/s3/chapter05.html)

Synchronize your breathing to create synergy for strength through the whole body. A movement pattern, pose or exercise strengthens your breath through movement first to send power through the nervous, neuromuscular and to and through the musculoskeletal system. This is strength and power. Breathing increases the nervous systems amplitude first. When you increase this amplitude you can transfer it through your musculoskeletal system. If you are not using your breath when training, you are not transferring power from the nervous system through the musculoskeletal system in an optimal nor in a functional way. You need to maintain the stability platform to move power form it, if not, it will be forced and strained and you will develop pain and injury and compensate your strength potential. Look at it like this, you cannot run I-tunes or Skype programs with first generation Microsoft Windows. You need an operating system that can run those programs effectively and properly; similarly to the body training only the musculoskeletal system. You need your breath and alignment to perform strength and training programs effectively, functionally and properly. Training just the musculoskeletal system is just like using the first generation of Microsoft Windows. It is very limited in what it can do today.

BREATHING AND STRENGTH EXERCISES

When you inhale and are waiting to punch, kick, jump or perform the next repetition in your strength or exercise routine, for example, you need the ability to keep recycling your breath, meaning the ability to inhale to have power for your exhalation for each repetition. Recycle your inhalation to have maximum power output in your exhalation. These exercises listed here are great for strengthening your breathing technique. I only added a handful but try and add the breathing technique to theses strength exercises. I added a diversity of exercises so you can see how the breathing technique works. I will publish more training materials for strength, power and performance. But, you need to be functional first.

- Kettlebell/Front Squat- Page 60, 61, 62
- Kettlebell/Dumbbell Press- Page 63, 64, 65
- Kettlebell Swing- Page 66, 67, 68
- Dead Lift- Page 69
- Push Up- Page 70
- Straight Back Sit Up- Page 71

Notice how your will muscles contract and stretch and how range of motion and flexibility improves instantly. As you inhale you will stabilize the abdominals with tension and pressure. And as you exhale hiss, the abdominals stay contracted isometrically. This allows you to maintain stability, alignment and power through your movements. Depending on the exercise depends on a longer, shorter or a pausing breathing cycle.

- A long breathing cycle is similar to running.
- A shorter breathing cycle is similar to a kettle bell swing.
- A pausing breathing cycle is more of a static hold at the end of press or a snatch.

BREATHING AND FLEXIBILITY EXERCISES

Once you have finished with Breathing and the Strength Exercises, try and add the breathing technique to these flexibility exercises listed. The breathing is similar but different than the strength exercises.

- Lunge - Page 73, 74
- Lying Down Knee Raise- Page 75
- One Arm Reach Spinal Side Bend- Page 76, 77
- Alternating High Knee Spinal Rotation- Page 78, 79

HOW TO USE THE BREATHING
CYCLE FOR FLEXIBILITY

The inhalation stabilizes the core and spine, contracts muscles to stabilize joints and loads the stretch. The exhalation releases the power through the mobility and movement. One breathing cycle is an inhalation and an exhalation.

In the first breathing cycle:
- Breathe in deep to stabilize the abdominals and bring power to the core.
- As you breathe in focus on contracting muscles to stabilize the joint's alignment first through the motion. Focus on inhaling and contracting muscles at the same time.
- Once you reach the point where the motion stops in the movement, hold the contraction and stretch for 3-5 seconds. You should be at the apex of the inhalation.
- Then from the held position, (Don't move back to the start. You will be in mid position.) exhale hiss into the motion but maintaining or increasing the muscular contraction through the movement or stretch. There should be more range of motion in the movement when you exhale. If not, feel for the ease of the position.

In the second breathing cycle:
- After the exhale hiss, you should have increased your range of motion. From this new position, breathe in again focusing on inhaling and contracting the same muscles. Notice if the breath gets longer and the contractions become stronger.
- Exhale hiss again into the motion, contracting and stretching those muscles while maintaining alignment. There should be more range of motion again in the movement when you exhale again. If not, feel for the ease of the position.

Perform this breathing technique for 3-5 breathing cycles in the movements. You can do more if you want. The first two cycles work at activating and integrating the circuitry. The next 2 to 3 cycles are when you start to feel the ease of the position and see the range of motion increase. If you have little to no motion, it's ok, keep working with the repetitions. I am more concerned about the breathing cycles (the inhalation connecting to the core and the muscular contractions and the exhalation producing stretch and motion) producing a neuromuscular pathway recognized by the brain for the musculoskeletal system to develop alignment and motion properly.

The breathing cycles are not meant to be done fast. The purpose is to:
- Contract muscles to maintain alignment through stability and produce flexibility and range of motion.
- Produce stamina in the pose and the motion.
- Synchronize and integrate all the systems together.

You now see why breathing is the most important thing for health, movement, power and strength. If you don't practice, you will produce a compensated subpar system.

Conclusion
"We are what we repeatedly do. Excellence, then, is not an act, but a habit." -Aristotle

When breathing is not function, it is not efficient nor effective. Therefore, compensation happens and alignment and movement become dysfunctional. When one joint or muscles is not strong or stable, then other joints and muscles make up for the weakness and lack of function. This tends to happen form sitting too much, isolated muscular strength training or training with poor stability and alignment.

The reason you need to train your breath to be functional is because the abdominals and the core provide stability to the spine. And, the hips need to be functional and balanced because their position provides alignment to the spine. How the hips are tilted, from front to back, will determine the spines position. The hips tilted forward hyperextends the spine. The hips tilted back, rounds the spine. This is the importance of gluteal strength: to keep the hips in a balanced aligned position. Alignment strengthens everything in the motion, where as misalignment only strengthens muscles maintaining misalignment. As strength goes up under misalignment, the imbalances get weaker and range of motion and mobility diminish. My book, *The Balanced Body*, teaches you more about how to correct and restore balance to your hips for optimal performance, to resolve pain and strain and prevent injury. It also helps to synchronize and train your breathing pattern through functional movement patterns to restore alignment and balance. Once the foundation is set, you can add weights to strengthen alignment and balance to be stronger. Think of alignment in the beginning as wood supporting and producing a foundation. As you increase the strength of alignment, its strength alchemizes into steel and so forth, becoming stronger and stronger over time.

Don't train misalignment and asymmetry; it will only work against you decreasing your mobility and range of motion. You can train the breathing pattern in all exercises like the chest press, lat pull, pull-up, dip, etc. Just use the breathing technique in the motion and you will feel the abdominals tighten and stabilize. What you are is what you train and what you train is what you strengthen and become.

Strength Exercises
Kettlebell/Front Squat

- You can perform this squat anyway you choose. It can be a front squat, etc.
- From the standing position, keep your feet straight or slightly turned out. Contract your quads and glutes in the standing position.
- Perform the bracing breath technique, inhaling through the nose and tightening the abdominals, as you squat to the floor.

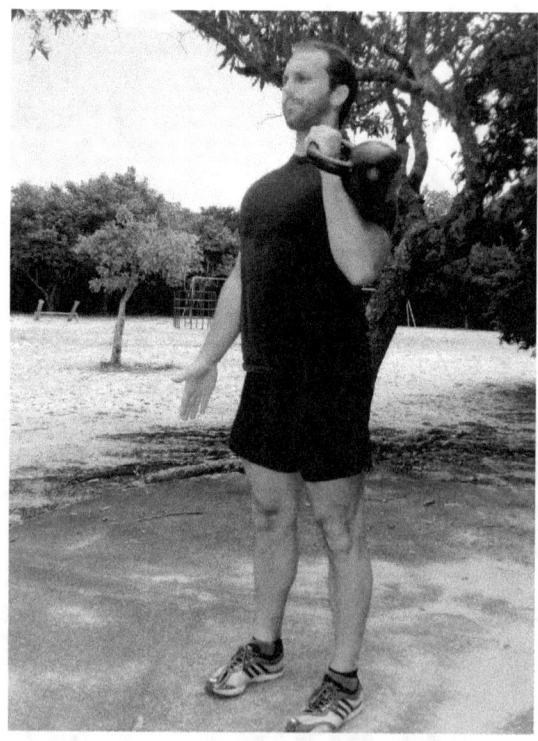

- First, focus on the abdominal tension using the bracing breath. This will produce the stability to keep the hips and spine straight in your squat, preventing the hips from rolling forward hyperextending the lumbar spine and from the hips rolling back rounding the thoracic spine. Preventing hyperextension and a rounded spine in your squat will make your legs stronger because of alignment. If you use the breathing technique correctly you will feel you abdominals become very tense.
- Exhale hiss (through pursed lips) the pressure from the inhalation and return to the standing position and contract the quads and glutes.

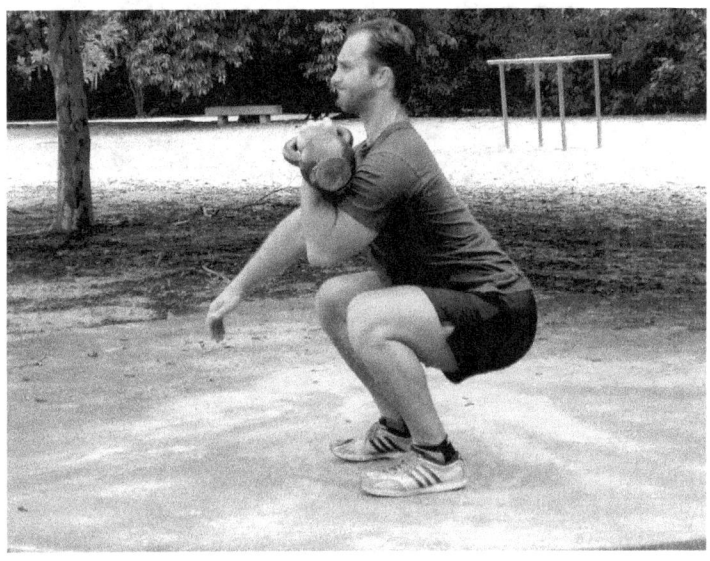

- Once the your squat becomes functional and the core is stabilizing the hips, abdominals and spine, you can begin to perform a deep-seated squat to the floor. You need the bracing breath to do this. And for this reason, for the hip and spine to maintain alignment. The hips should not roll or tilt back rounding the spine in your squat; this is compensation.

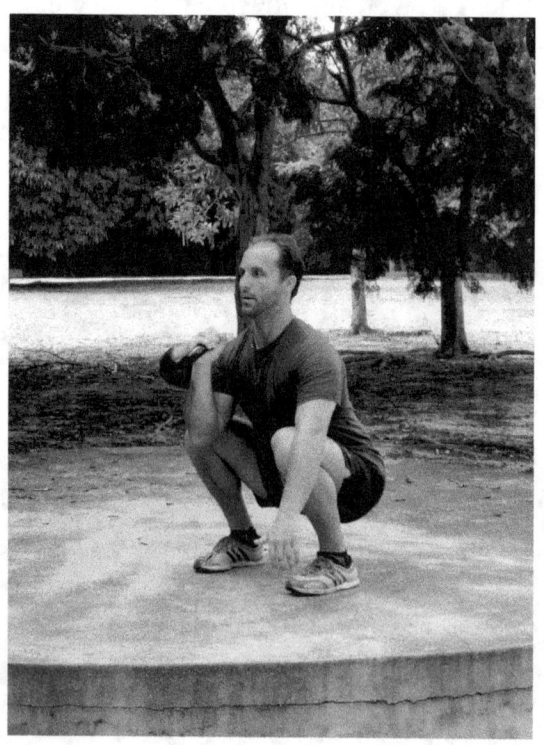

Kettlebell/Dumbbell Press

- You can perform this press from the lunge, seated or standing position.
- Pull your elbow into your ribcage to begin the loading phase.
- Breathe in through the nose performing the bracing breath technique.

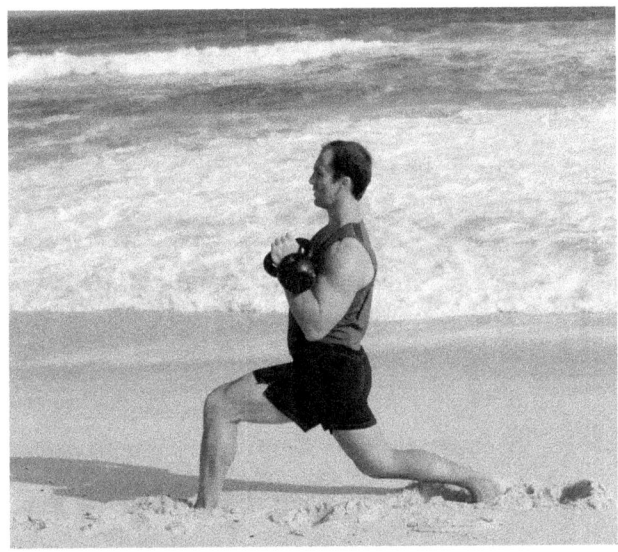

- Once you have the breath loaded from the inhalation, squeeze your glutes, exhale hiss and press the weight above your head. As you press you will strengthen the core.

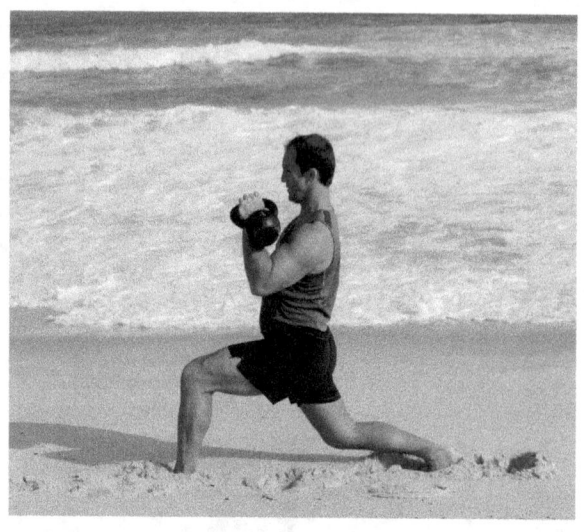

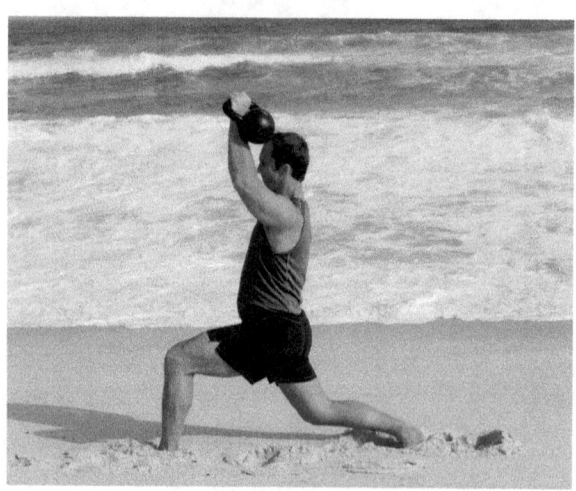

- The harder you exhale hiss through pursed lips, the more abdominal tension you use to press.

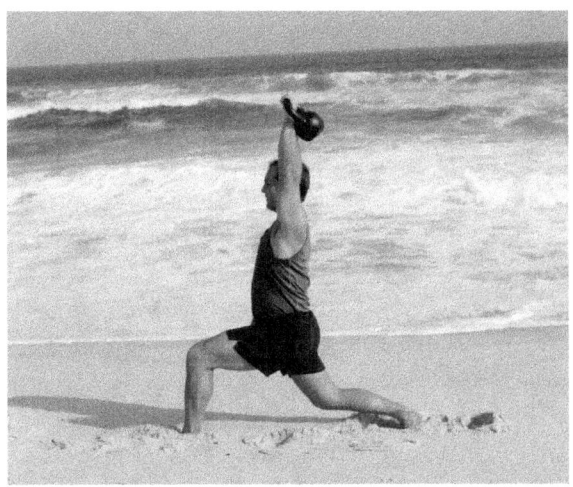

- Inhale to stabilize and brace the abdominals as you lower the weight back to the start position. Exhale hiss to do another rep.

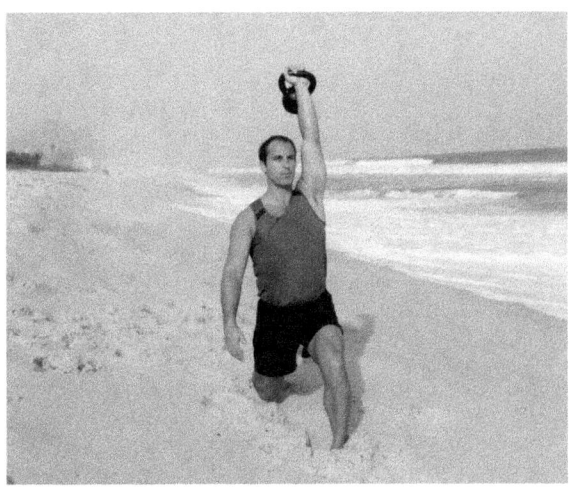

Kettlebell Swing

- Great exercise for strengthening your breathing performance.
- On the swing back of the bell, inhale through the nose using the bracing technique.
- Keep the knees bent and stretch the hamstrings.

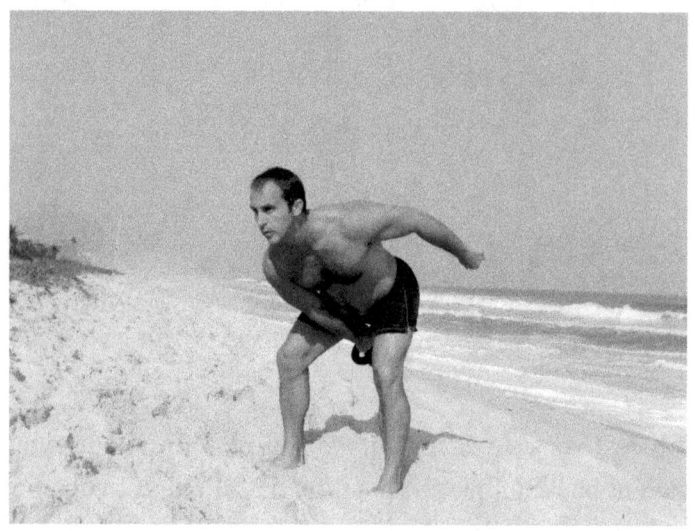

- Exhale hiss through pursed lips and drive the bell up to chest height. When the bell reaches the top, in the standing position, contract the quads and the glutes.

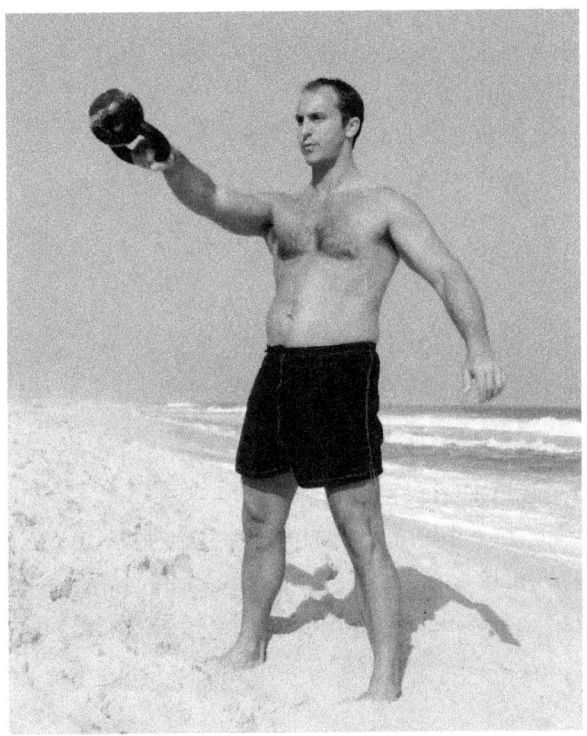

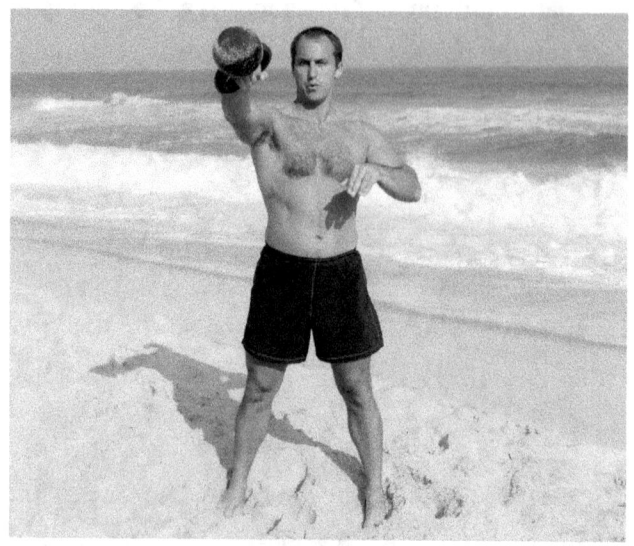

- Keep your grip tight on the bell and your lat muscles (back muscles on the side) tight as well.
- Inhale again using the bracing breath technique to lower the bell down to load your swing and exhale hiss to dive the bell up and squeeze the quads and glutes at the top for the split second before the next rep.

Please learn how to do the swing properly from a professional before you attempt to try this exercise.

Dead Lift

- If you have a problem with your kettle bell swing, learn to dead lift effectively first. The breathing is the same as the kettle bell swing. Inhale through the nose using the bracing breath technique to pick up the weight.

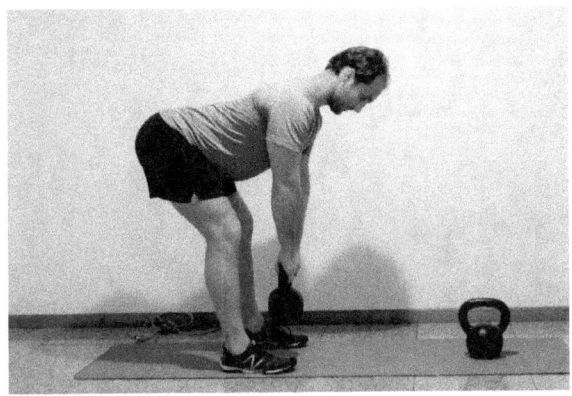

- Exhale hiss and lift the weight up to the standing position and squeeze the quads and glutes in the standing position. Perform slowly. Focus on stretching the hamstrings. Perform desired number of reps.

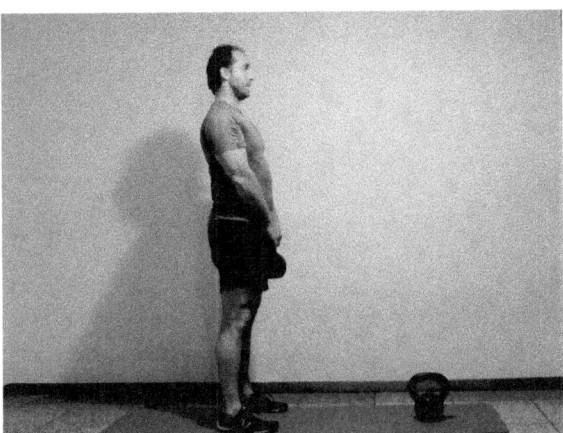

Push Up

- Contract your glutes and quads.
- Breathe in through the nose using the bracing breath technique and lower yourself down to the floor.

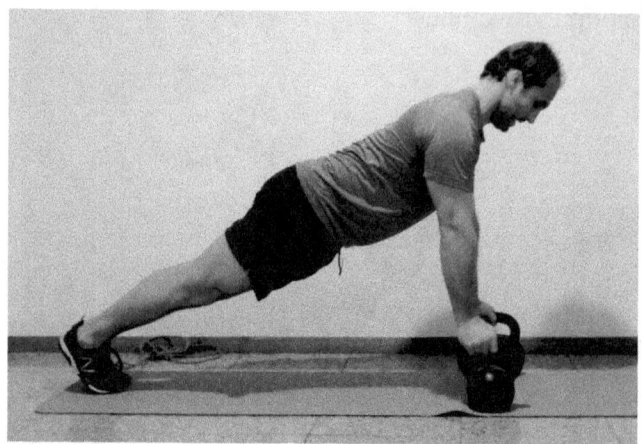

- When you reach the floor, exhale hiss through pursed lips and push yourself back up to the start position. During your repetitions, keep your glutes and quads contracted when moving up and down to preserve alignment of the hips.

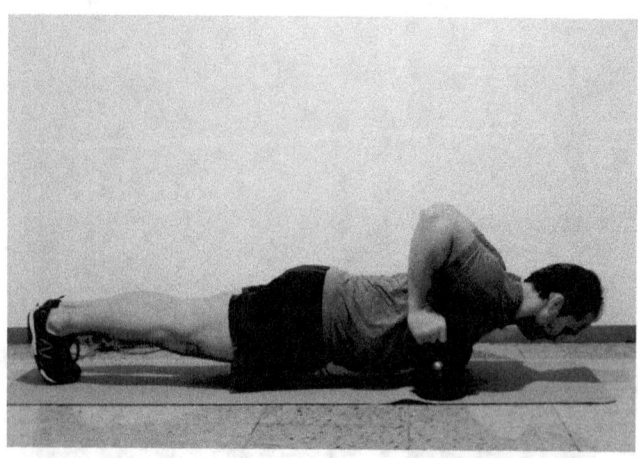

Straight Back Sit Up

- Lying on your back with your knees up and feet flat on the floor, breathe in using the bracing breath technique and lift your back off the floor.

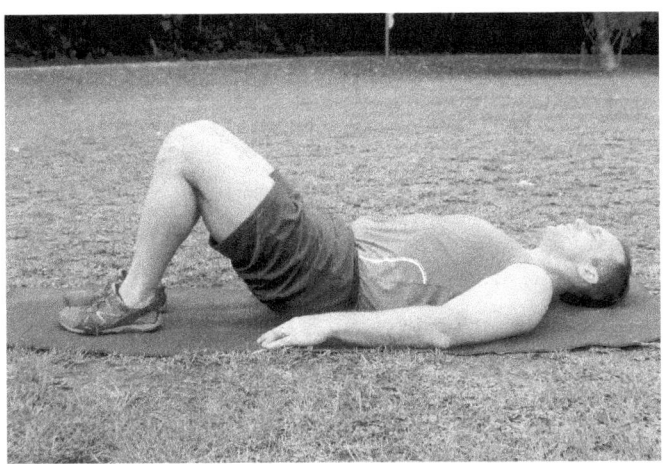

- When you lift your back off the floor, don't do a crunch. Lift up, hold and focus on pulling the shoulders back. Maintain spine alignment.

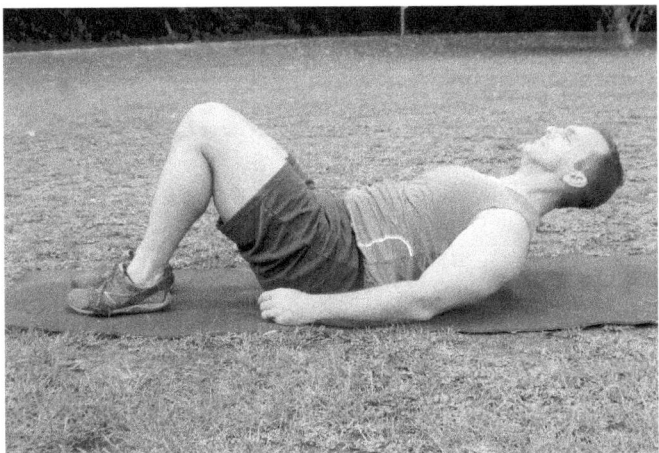

- Exhale hiss and lower to the floor.
- You can do the breathing the opposite way if you like as well. I breathe in as I lift up because if I want to add motion to this

position, like a rotation, I am ready to perform and move on the exhalation.

Flexibility Exercises
Lunge

- Assume the lunge position with one leg forward and the other back. Make sure the feet are straight.
- Contract the glute on the leg that is back. Keep the leg straight in the lunge. You can contract the quads as well but focus on the glutes first.

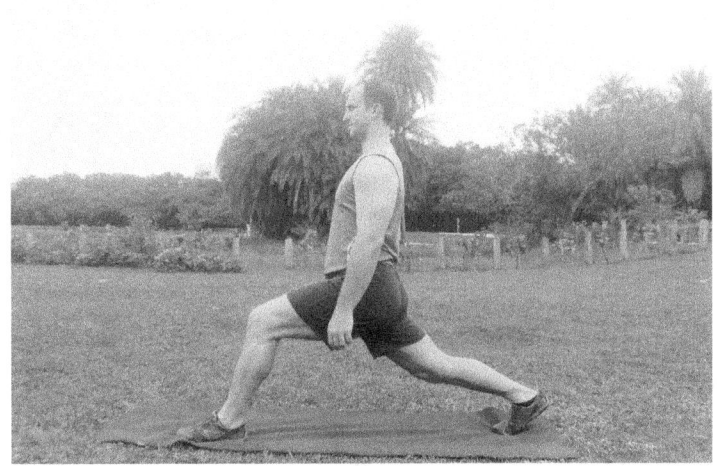

- Breathe in and lower your hips down to the floor maintaing the glute/quad contraction. As you lower the hips down to the floor, keep contratcing the glute to stabilize the hip. You will feel the hip flexor stretch.

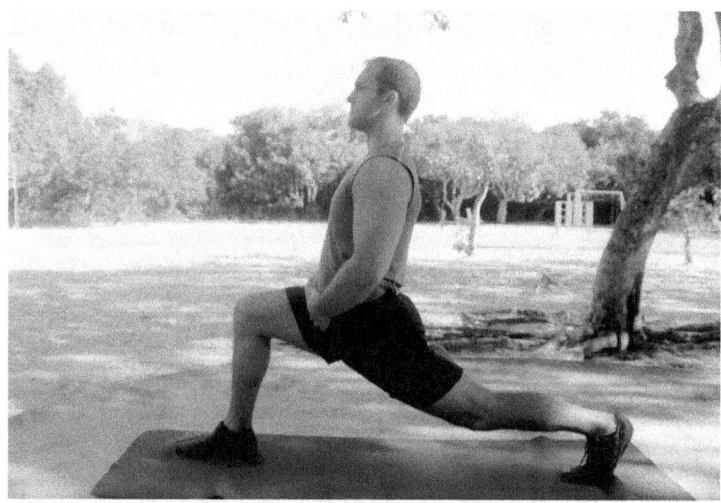

- When the motion stops as well as the inhalation, hold the position and exhale hiss from this positon and see if there is more motion on the exhale. Breathe in again maintaining the glute and quad contraction from the lower position and then exhale hiss and try to lower further naturally.
- Reapeat for 3 to 5 breathing cycles and then switch sides.

Lying Down Knee Raise Leg Extension

- Breathe in and lift your knee up toward your chest using the bracing breath technique.

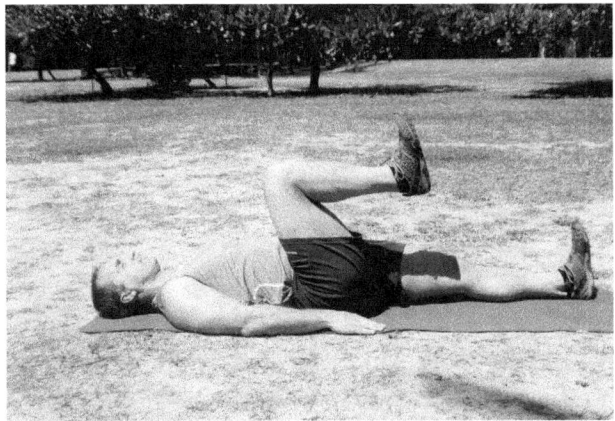

- Exhale hiss and straighten the leg contracting the quads and slightly pull the toes toward the knee. This will produce core stability and the reciprocation for the contraction of the quads to stretch the hamstrings.

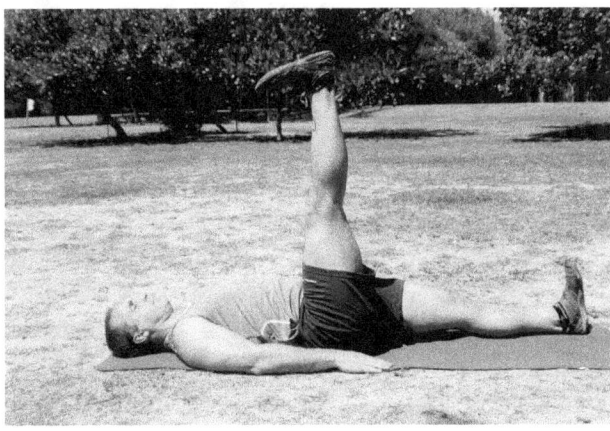

- Breathe in and bend the knee and see if it is easier to lift the knee higher toward the chest.
- Repeat for 3-5 breathing cycles and perform the other side.

Standing Side Bend One Arm Reach

- From the standing position spread the feet shoulder width apart. Contract the glutes and quads and reach one arm up above your head. This will ground your movement.

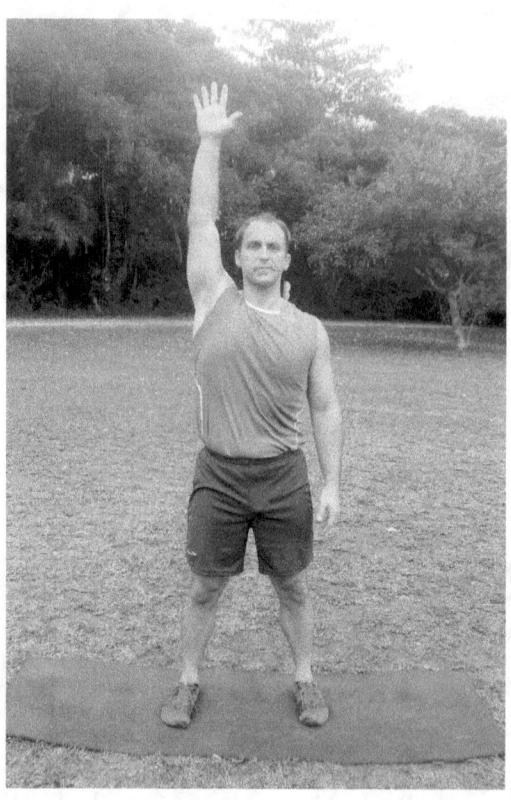

- Breathe in and stretch the arm that is up to the side. Keep the abdominals, obliques, lats, quads and glutes tight when bending from this platform. Contract the lat and oblique on the side the arm is down. When the motion stops as well as the inhalation, exhale hiss and see if there is more motion in the stretch.
- Continue for 3-5 breathing cycles in the side bend contracting and reaching. Exhale hiss and move back to the center. Perform on the other side.

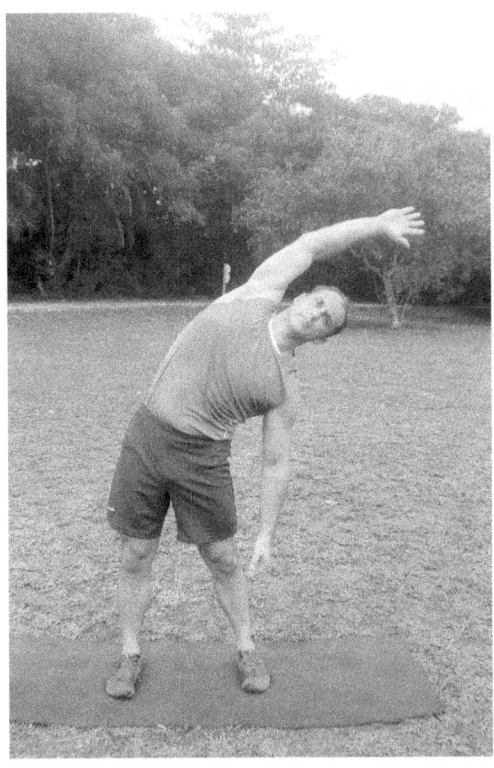

Alternate High Kneeling Spinal Rotation

- Place your arms in front of you.
- Contract the glutes.

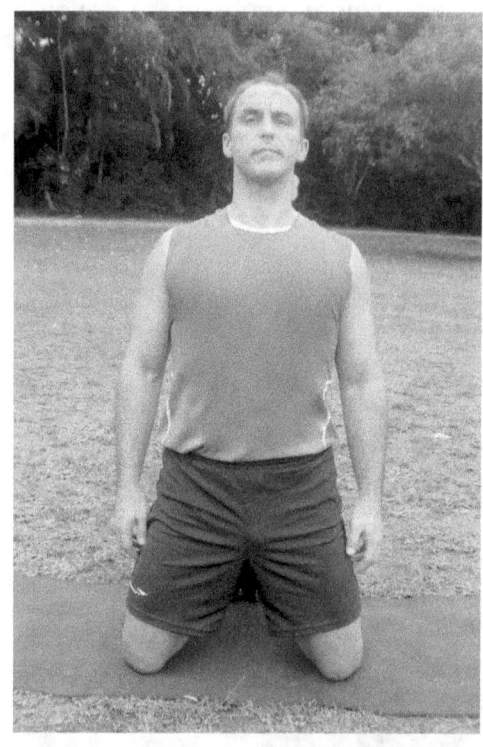

- Breathe in and rotate the spine to one side, contracting the oblique and the opposite side lat. Do not try to rotate too much. Just let your brain feel the muscles contract to guide the motion. Once they can guide the motion, you will improve range of motion.
- Perform 3-5 breathing cycles in the rotation with the contraction of the lat and opposite side oblique while keeping the glutes contracted to maintain alignment and balance of the hips for the spine.
- After 3-5 breathing cycles, exhale hiss back to the center and perform the other side.

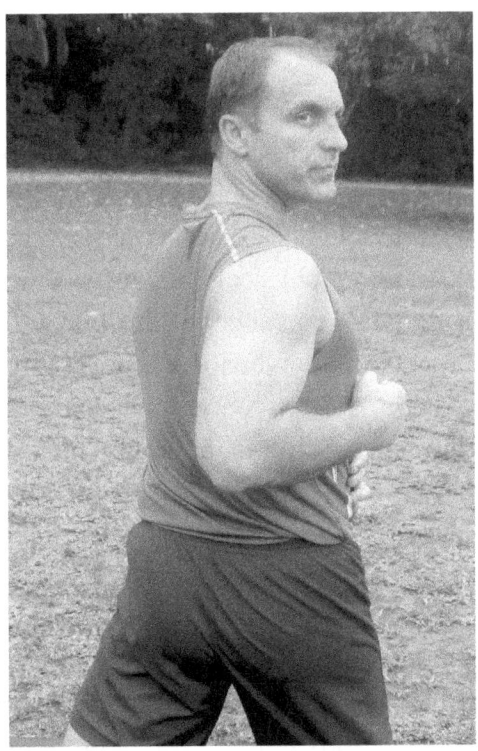

About the Author

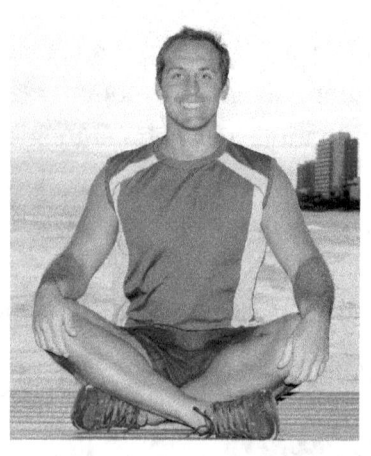 Jason Kelly graduated from Temple University in Exercise Science. He has been an exercise physiologist and massage therapist for over 19 years. He has worked with diabetes and cardiovascular disease programing; the geriatric, general and athletic populations designing prevention and strength programs; corporations teaching their employees how to stay healthy, breathe, move, exercise well and use better ergonomics in the workplace.

As a fitness director he taught, strength, power and health comes from within; how you function to move, not just move. With this philosophy, he overhauled the entire program in the fitness facility with his functional mindset and approach that had instant success and results. He has taught workshops to physical therapists, athletic trainers and massage therapists and to the general population.

From working with a diversity of populations, he saw that prevention is rarely taught and misconceptions are widely accepted and used leading to high statistics of pain, injury, disease and disorder. Incorporating his years of skill and experience, he developed the *Breathe, Stabilize, Move-Function First Method* to combat and resolve pain, injury, disease and disorders like musculoskeletal ones and for people to move well, freely and frequently for longevity. When you are functional, have alignment and breathe well, you move well developing prevention, health, fitness or strength in your life or sport. It does not matter who you are, young, old, athlete or not, you need to be functional first to have the shield of prevention and the balanced foundation to nurture movement and foster strength to cultivate their growth.